DEATH STALKS THE YAKAMA

DEATH STALKS THE YAKAMA

Epidemiological Transitions and Mortality On the Yakama Indian Reservation, 1888-1964

CLIFFORD E. TRAFZER

MICHIGAN STATE UNIVERSITY PRESS

EAST LANSING

Michigan State University Press, East Lansing, Michigan, USA, 48823-5202

Library of Congress Cataloging-in-Publication Data

Trafzer, Clifford E.
 Death stalks the Yakama : epidemiological transitions and mortality on
the Yakama Indian reservation, 1888—1964 / Clifford E. Trafzer
  p. cm.
 Includes bibliographical references and index.
 ISBN 0-87013-463-9
 1. Yakama Indians—Mortality—Statistics. 2.Yakama children—
Mortality—Statistics. 3.Yakama children—Diseases—Statistics. 4.
Yakama children—Nutrition—Statistics. 6. Yakama Indian Reservation
(Wash.)—Statistics, Vital. I.Title.
E99.Y2T73 1997
304.6'4'089974—dc21   96-52172
                   CIP

06 05 04 03 02 01 00 99 98 97 1 2 3 4 5 6 7 8 9 10

This study was made possible in part through funding provided
by the American Council of Learned Societies, the Phillips
Fund of the American Philosophical Society, National
Endowment for the Humanities, Newberry Library,
Rockefeller Foundation, and the University of California,
Riverside.

All royalties from the publication of this book will be contributed to the Maternal Child Health Department of the Yakama
Nation for prenatal, infant, and children's care.

This book is respectfully dedicated to Yakama children who suffered the wrath of disease on the reservation and to their parents who mourned their deaths. It is also dedicated to my own children, Tess Nashone, Hayley Kachine, and Tara Tsaile who have not had to face the devastation of pneumonia, heart disease, tuberculosis, whooping cough, and other diseases that killed so many native children in the recent past.

CONTENTS

Preface
ix

Part One
Introduction
1

Part Two
The Yakama
23

Part Three
Yakama Death Certificates: Theoretical
and Methodological Orientations
67

Part Four
Comparison of Yakama Death
Rates with Other Populations
123

Part Five
Conclusion
187

Appendix
212

Bibliography
241

Index
267

PREFACE

The present work is an outgrowth of my previous research on various Indian tribes living on the Columbia River Plateau. In 1977, I began research on a book dealing with the history of the Palouse Indians of eastern Washington. During the course of my research, I traveled west with my colleague, Richard D. Scheuerman, to the Yakama Reservation where we interviewed descendants of the Palouse people. As a result, we met Mary Jim and Andrew George, and our association with these and other elders enriched our research and our lives. This was my first acquaintance with the Yakama Reservation, and it is one that has developed over the years. In addition to researching on the reservation, I traveled to Seattle to conduct research at the National Archives, Pacific Northwest Region. There I met the gracious and helpful archivist, Joyce Justice, who introduced me to the papers of the Yakama Indian Agency, and I was impressed with the large collection of materials available dealing with the Yakama Reservation. After becoming acquainted with the collection, I determined that when I finished the Palouse book, I would begin a study of the Yakama Reservation. In 1986, Washington State University Press published *Renegade Tribe: The Palouse Indians and the Invasion of the Inland Pacific Northwest,* and after the book was released, I started work on a study of the Yakama Reservation.

Originally, I intended to write a history of the Yakama Reservation, and I began reading the letters found in the voluminous letter books kept at the National Archives. However, the more I read, the more I realized that the Yakama Reservation was little different from other reservations in terms of administrative history. I asked Joyce Justice if I could review some other documents, including records of the Indian court, birth records, death certificates, bills of sale, and marriage certificates. These were documents that required a statistical methodology, and I resolved to collect these documents in order to study selected aspects of Yakama social history.

I first worked through the bills of sale, since I had a good deal of experience dealing with the Indian trade on another reservation. After coding the bills of sale and entering them into the computer, I generated data that demonstrated the purchasing power of Yakama women on the reservation. The results of this work have been published in Nancy Shoemaker, editor, *Negotiators of Change: Historical Perspectives on Native American Women*, Routledge, 1995. Work on the Yakama bills of sale and helpful encouragement from Fred Hoxie stimulated my interest in the social history of the people, and so I turned my attention to nearly four thousand Yakama Death Certificates in Record Group 75 of the National Archives, Pacific Northwest Region.

When I was a child, my mother explained that Indian reservations had been dangerous places to live, places where large numbers of people, particularly small children, died because of diseases. This is a common theme among Indian people and among historians who study Native Americans. I decided to investigate the notion through a statistical analysis of Yakama Death Certificates. I chose to focus on one reservation, knowing that no one had used Death Certificates in work on Yakama people. In order to study disease, population, and childhood mortality on the Yakama Indian Reservation, I copied every Death Certificate available, sorted the documents to remove duplicates, and arranged them by year. Next, the certificates were coded and entered into the computer. With the able help of Neal Hickman, Department of Sociology, University of California, Riverside, and currently Director of Research for the Gallop Organization, we generated a great deal of data dealing with causes of death, ages at death, and location of the the person at the time of death. We addressed a number of variables and asked numerous questions about the data. Hickman's assistance has been invaluable. For eight years I have labored with the data and have written a narrowly-defined scholarly study emphasizing on aspects of death on the Yakama Indian Reservation using an interdisciplinary Native American studies approach. I focus on epidemiological and nutritional transitions among the Yakama that significantly affected disease and death on the reservation over time.

Work on Native American mortality has been difficult personally due to the deaths of so many people, particularly infants and children. People of the Confederated Tribes of the Yakama Nation are more than numbers to me, and the undertaking challenged my ability to work with the data. However, the study of death on the Yakama Reservation is an important project in Native American history, and I felt it deserved discussion, analysis, and interpretation. I trust this study will encourage other scholars to use Death Certificates available for other reservations in their epidemiological studies of diverse Native American populations. I urge scholars to compare their data with Yakama statistics. It is hoped that scholars will examine the reservation system using the voluminous documents kept in the National Archives that lend themselves to statistical approaches and isolate epidemiological and nutritional areas of historical inquiry. Russell Thornton, Gregory Campbell, Cheryl Howard, Robert Boyd, Matthew Snipp, Henry Dobyns, and other scholars have worked in this area of study for years, and we need to build on their good work. In particular, I hope that this book will prompt other scholars to create their own "grassroots" data bases rather than rely on those created by the Census Bureau or presented in the Annual Reports of the Commissioner of Indian Affairs. While it is true that more time and energy are required to create new databases from Death Certificates, Birth Certificates, and Tribal Censuses for individual reservations, it is equally true that the benefits of these for the study of Indian people will be great.

Creation of a new Native American history centered on epidemiology, nutrition, and public health will provide an opportunity for comparative analysis regarding death on various reservations. The data presented in this study is on file in the Department of History and Native American Studies Program, University of California, Riverside, and I invite scholars to contact me regarding the data and the results of this study. I hope my research will further the study of Native Americans and will be of practical use to the Indian people living on the Yakama Reservation who will have an historical source analyzing mortality on the reservation during the early twentieth century. This might be of singular importance to anyone wishing to examine the significance of the Hanford Nuclear Plant on the health of Yakama people since the 1940s or the importance of suicide as a cause of death prior to 1964. Drafts of this study have been shared with members of the Yakama Nation, and copies of the work are on file at the Yakama Tribal Library, Yakima Indian Health Center, Washington Center for Health Statistics, and Washington Governor's Office of Indian Affairs.

Several people have been instrumental in the preparation of this project. Neal Hickman deserves much credit for helping me analyze and understand the data. Helen Schuster provided the fieldwork that is the basis for the cultural presentations of death on the reservation and read the manuscript. I sincerely appreciate all that she has done to further the study of Yakama people. I am indebted to Eugene S. Hunn and James Selam for producing a unique and powerful book on the mid-Columbia tribes. Also, Hunn read and reviewed the manuscript, offering insightful revisions that improved the work. His letter to me is a wealth of information, and I thank him for taking the time to help me. Similar gratitude is extended to John R. Weeks of San Diego State University for reading and commenting on the manuscript. His constructive criticisms benefited me greatly, as did his introduction to me of works by two important scholars.

The research of Abdel Omran and Barry Popkin, both of the University of North Carolina, changed the way I thought about and approached my data in terms of epidemiology as significant factors in Yakama history. I also thank Robert Boyd for his magnificent work on infectious diseases among Northwestern Indians in the eighteenth and nineteenth centuries. I thank Kirsten Holm of the Center for Health Statistics, Department of Health, in Washington state for her information on the registry of past Death Certificates. My sincere thanks also is extended to Howard Kushner of San Diego State University and the University of California, San Diego, who read portions of the manuscript and offered criticism relative to diet, nutrition, foods, and mortality. Terry Smith, Lisa Firth, John Moran, and Brad Richie are all physicians or health officials who read portions of the manuscript and commented on clinical and medical explanations of death.

I am grateful to the faculty of the History and Ethnic Studies departments at the University of California, Riverside, who have been so supportive of Indian people, Native American Studies, and my own work. I wish to thank my colleagues Gene Anderson, Ed Butler, Carl Cranor, Ralph Crowder, Jim Erickson, Bob Griffin, Bernd Magnus, Armando Navarro, Raymond Orbach, Steffi San Buenaventura, Carol Shammas, Sterling Stuckey, Carlos Vélez-Ibáñez, and David Warren. I thank other scholars for reading and commenting on the manuscript, including Thomas Avramis, Thomas Clark, James Sandos, and Richard Scheuerman. I offer a special thanks to Roy Richie of the Huntington Library who, years ago, encouraged me to concentrate on social history and complete this work, and to John Moran of the Yakama Indian Health Center in Toppenish, and Rosalie Aleck of the Maternal Child Health Program who helped to make this contribution to the people. Native American scholars have been supportive of this work, including Kimberly Blaeser, Edward Castillo, Jeanette Costo, Brenda Child, Cheryl Duran, Lee Francis, Rebecca Kugle, Sandy Lynch, Louis Owens, Georges E. Sioui, Gerald Vizenor, Donna Whitt, and Loretta Winters.

I also express my gratitude to Joyce Justice of the National Archives, Pacific Northwest Region, Myra Andersen of the University of California, Riverside, Tomas Rivera Library, Colleen Veomett of the Yakama Nation Tribal Library, and John Guido of Washington State University Holland Library. The editors on the Michigan State University Press staff also deserve my sincere appreciation for helping shape and present this work.

Most of all, I thank Lee Ann for her encouragement, patience, and advice. My children, Tess, Hayley, and Tara, have been understanding of the time I have spent away from them while researching and writing this work. Finally, I pay tribute to the people living on the Yakama Reservation, people who have survived and grown in strength despite depression, disease, and death. The Yakama have emerged a strong confederated Indian nation that has never forgotten its traditional roots. I hope that my work will be of use to the people of the Yakama Nation.

Clifford E. Trafzer
Yucaipa, California
March 1997

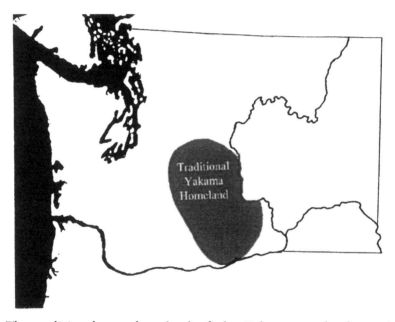

The traditional core homeland of the Yakama people shown in relation to boundaries of the present-day State of Washington.

PART ONE

INTRODUCTION

Death Stalks the Yakama reflects my interest in an interdisciplinary approach to Native American history, using documents and methodologies of social history, religious studies, anthropology, sociology, oral history, and oral literature. It is hoped that this approach contributes to scholarly inquiry about native peoples by offering a broader understanding of the statistical data created from the Yakama Death Certificates.[1] The book is intended to be a narrowly defined scholarly study that focuses primarily, but not exclusively, on Death Certificates, Death Registers, and Birth Registers. The work is not a demographic or population history of the Yakama, but a study of epidemiological transitions as they relate to death on one reservation for seventy-six years—from 1888 to 1964. There is no pretense that this is the definitive work on epidemiology as it relates to death on the Yakama Reservation, but epidemiological transition is used as the theoretical backdrop and conceptual context for much of what happened to the tribes and bands that made up the Yakama Nation during the early twentieth century.

The theoretical framework used in the presentation of the Yakama death data is derived from the work of Abdel R. Omran and Barry Popkin. Omran offers the theory and provides a model

1

that informs us about Yakama epidemiological transitions. He argues that in the United States, there was an historical shift in the nineteenth century from "pandemics of infectious diseases to the degenerative and man-made diseases which are now the chief forms of illness and causes of death."[2] He maintains that the initial decline in mortality in the United States was more a function of "improvements in living standards and changes in the nature of some diseases" than it was from "medical progress, widespread sanitation, or organized health services."[3] In part this was true for Yakama people whose standard of living improved as a result of wage earning during World War II and as a result of federal and tribal programs emerging out of the Indian New Deal of the 1930s and 1940s.

The Yakama benefited significantly during that era from advances in public health, medical advancements, better sanitation, new housing, and sanitation-isolation programs designed to destroy tuberculosis. They also benefited from a natural decline in tuberculosis, a disease that seems to have run its course within the population by the late 1940s or early 1950s. Thus, Omran's theory of epidemiological transitions reveals much about infectious diseases, health, and historical eras. He asserts that the transition from high to low mortality derives from "a combination of medical developments," including the introduction of antibiotics, sanitation, and public medical health care. He also argues that there are fixed periods of time when "Old World" epidemics of smallpox, measles, fevers, influenza, typhoid, tuberculosis, and cholera are "replaced by heart diseases, cancer, stroke, diabetes, gastric ulcer . . . together with increased mental illness, accidents, [and] disease due to industrial exposure."[4]

Omran argues that generally "mortality patterns distinguish three major successive stages of epidemiological transition including the Age of Pestilence and Famine, the Age of Receding Pandemics, and the Age of Degenerative and Man-Made Diseases."[5] Yakama epidemiological history began with the pre-contact period when there was no solid data recorded. Even before the arrival of Meriwether Lewis and William Clark in 1805, Yakama people began to enter the Age of Pestilence as Euro-American traders introduced infectious diseases to Native Americans living along the coast of the Pacific Northwest.[6] Thus, throughout the entire nineteenth and early twentieth centuries, the Yakama lived in the Age of Pestilence, facing the scourge of many contagious diseases. During the twentieth century this age continued as tuberculosis, pneumonia, gastrointestinal disorders, influenza, and other diseases preyed on the Yakama population. By the late nineteenth century, smallpox had declined significantly as a killer of American Indians. However, in 1900, a total of 30 native people living on the Yakama Reservation contracted smallpox and two of them died. Still, the disease was short lived on the reservation for no deaths due to smallpox were reported in 1901.[7] The Age of Pestilence and the Age of Receding Pandemics merged during the 1920s and 1930s, giving way to the Age of Degenerative and Man-Made Diseases. The watershed in Yakama epidemiological history was World War II, when tuberculosis, gastrointestinal disorders, and influenza declined. During the late 1940s and throughout the 1950s, man-made degenerative causes of death, including heart disease, cancer, and accidental deaths, became the leading causes of mortality among the Yakama.

Epidemiological transitions are greatly influenced by nutritional and dietary changes, a theory advanced by Barry Popkin who argues that there are predictable changes in diet that accompany modernization and result in new causes of death. The importance of nutrition as a precondition influencing deaths by certain diseases has also been advanced by Thomas McKeown and his associates. In his own words, McKeown argues that "the slow growth of the human population before the eighteenth century was due mainly to lack of food, and the rapid increase from that time resulted largely from improved nutrition."[8] For the Yakama, this occurred with white resettlement of Indian lands in the nineteenth and early twentieth centuries and with the changes that emerged during World War II when Yakama served as soldiers and defense workers. Diets changed and nutritional values of many refined foods were far less nutritious than traditional Indian foods. No longer did Yakama people eat roots, berries, game, and fish. After the 1930s, they primarily ate refined foods high in calories, cholesterol, carbohydrates, sugar, and saturated fats, purchased with cash they earned from wage labor, miscellaneous employment, the sale of livestock-agricultural products, and leases to non-Indians in the Yakima Valley. Ann G. Carmichael has pointed out that "biochemists contend that being under-nourished does not make the human body prone to more severe or more frequent infection, but biochemical models do not address the social circumstances which allow widespread under nutrition." She argues that "impoverished environment enhances morbidity and mortality" because "poorly nourished individuals rapidly exhaust protein and caloric reserves in the process of fighting infection." She demonstrates that poverty creates a situation in which infection is enhanced.[9] Susan Cotts Watkins and Etienne van de Walle also point out that "mortality may be tied to the availability of food at levels of under nourishment that fall short of starvation."[10] The link between disease and food was advanced by Thomas McKeown in *The Modern Rise of Population*, but his theory is refuted by other scholars, including S. Ryan Johansson. The importance of nutrition and the destruction of Yakama native foods are themes developed in this volume, but not at the expense of several other factors that influenced mortality. Clearly, public health, sanitation, housing, medical care, medicines, food, and anomie all played a role in Yakama mortality, and there is no intent here to privilege one factor over the other. All of them influenced the course of Yakama mortality history, but themes found in the works of Omran and Popkin relate to the Yakama situation during the late nineteenth and early twentieth centuries, and epidemiological transitions are the theoretical bases of this study.[11]

The destruction of native food resources on the Columbia Plateau as a result of white farming, ranching, and development is easy to document, but it is difficult to assess the biological effects of this historical transition during the late nineteenth and early twentieth centuries among Native Americans. People who once ate large quantities of roots, berries, fish, and game found their resources dwindling due to development and government policies that encouraged them to remain on the reservation to farm and ranch. In their ground-breaking study, *Fatal Years: Child Mortality in Late Nineteenth-Century America*, Samuel H. Preston and Michael R. Haines maintain that child mortality in 1900 was not linked to food because food was abundant and cheap.[12] Their statement pertained to America as a whole, but it surely did not apply to most Native Americans, particularly those living on the Yakama Reservation. Certainly, as Popkin has suggested, the destruction of native food resources had some impact on the health of the people, especially when the people lost their native foods and received no supplements to replace them in their diets. And even if they had received new foods of equal nutritional value, there is little reason to assume that their bodies could have biologically absorbed the full nutritive value of the food. Also, traditional native foods were (and are) far more than items to consume, for they were part of the sacred creation and were eaten ceremoniously during the year as part of religious ritual. The destruction of native plants and animals and the destruction of land forms through construction and development had a profound spiritual and psychological impact on native people as well as biological influences. This is not to argue that the loss of native foods was the only factor influencing death on the Yakama Reservation or that it was the most important condition surrounding death. It was one of many factors that influenced mortality on the reservation, factors born of policies and actions out of the control of native peoples.

All of the elements surrounding mortality on the Yakama Reservation, including the destruction of food resources, are difficult to quantify, but we know they influenced mortality on the reservation throughout the twentieth century. As a result of the destruction of food resources, white invasion, treaty making, the Plateau Indian War, political subjugation, Christian conversions, forced removal, relocation, and the reservation system, Indians living on the Yakama Reservation suffered a social anomie or depression that contributed to ill health and death. They also experienced the ill effects of having no public health program on the reservation, a concept that was in its infancy in the early twentieth century throughout the United States. The absence of public health contributed to deaths, particularly those resulting from infectious diseases such as tuberculosis, pneumonia, influenza, and gastrointestinal disorders. Public health and its significance in controlling disease was a new concept, and American Indians had little knowledge of public health initiatives. Gaining such information was complicated by two factors. Indians living on the Yakama Reservation spoke several dialects of three distinct language families, and English was not their primary (or perhaps even their secondary) language. And even if they spoke some English, many could not read printed information in English regarding issues of public health. Furthermore, public health educational programs among Native Americans were few, because the Office of Indian Affairs lacked sufficient funds to develop such programs. For their part, the Office of Indian Affairs offered some programs to encourage public health, particularly those involving mothers and their babies. Yet, such programs were small in nature, involving only a few people, and they did not have a great impact on mortality on the reservation.

Indians living on the Yakama Reservation had little knowledge of sanitation or the use of soap and water to kill germs on one's body, clothing, plates, cups, or eating utensils. Native peoples did not understand the dangers of sharing such material items or passing a pipe of tobacco from one person to the next. They did not know the dangers of giving away such items after a person died. Among native peoples living on the Yakama Reservation, giveaways after the death of a person were the "law." It was a practice established at the time of creation, and it was unthinkable not to pass along to the living the clothing, blankets, bedding, pots, pans, pipes, weapons, and other personal items of the dead. Bacteria spread in this manner, infecting and killing others through the transfer of diseases. Dangerous bacteria also traveled through unprotected foods, dust from dirt floors, and soiled bandages used to cover open wounds on the neck resulting from scrofula (lymphatic tuberculosis).

Native Americans from the Yakama Reservation lived in substandard housing with dirt floors, no running water, and poor ventilation. When people became ill from infectious diseases, women usually took care of them within the home. Patients with infectious diseases were not isolated from other members of the family. Some of these diseases, most importantly tuberculosis, developed slowly and were hard to detect without medical expertise. Doctors, nurses, hospitals, clinics, and sanitoria were few or non-existent throughout the twentieth century. Native Americans had little or no understanding of these infectious diseases, maladies little understood by medical doctors or the general public of the United States in the early twentieth century. As a result of all of these factors, Indians died on the Yakama Reservation, particularly infants.

Statistical data from Death Registers and Certificates recording mortality among the Yakama between 1888 and 1923 is poor, but this data is included in the study because it is part of the total data available from Death Registers and Certificates. The data for Yakama mortality from 1924 to 1964 is particularly strong and provides a unique opportunity to study Yakama

Indian social history during the early twentieth century (figure 1.1). All of the death data presented in this volume offer clinical explanations of death, not medical explanations. Medical doctors practicing on the Yakama Reservation and in the Yakima County Coroner's Office performed few autopsies on Yakama people, so few medical explanations of the cause of death are recorded on Yakama Death Certificates. Brad Richie, a medical doctor practicing at a Kaiser facility in Riverside, California, explained that this distinction is significant in the medical community. When it was pointed out that 71 percent of all cancer deaths among Yakama in this study were suffered by women and that uterine, cervical, breast, and stomach cancers were the major types of cancer, Richie responded by saying that doctors who were making these identifications could not have known for certain the differences among various reproductive system cancers without an autopsy. Furthermore, only a medical explanation of death could have confirmed that a person who had suffered for years from tuberculosis died of the disease rather than pneumonia that had invaded the body of the weakened patient. No autopsies appear in the Health and Hospital Records of the Yakama found in the National Archives, Pacific Northwest Region, and there are no indications on the Death Certificates that doctors performed any autopsies. Therefore, the data is limited to clinical explanations of death.

In spite of the limitations of clinical explanations of death, Professor James Sandos of the University of Redlands recently pointed out that clinical explanations of death are historically valuable. He offered as an example the many deaths of AIDS patients due to causes other than AIDS. Many HIV infected patients today die of pneumonia or other infectious diseases, not AIDS. The medical explanation of the cause of death might be, for example, pneumonia, which actually killed the person, but the underlying cause of death was the HIV virus that so weakened the individual that he or she became a perfect host for pneumonia which killed the person. Thus, a clinical and common-sense description of this cause of death would be the HIV virus, while the medical explanation would be pneumonia. Clinical explanations of causes of death, therefore, have value in any discussion of mortality, and these descriptions of death are the only ones available to scholars studying Yakama people. The analysis of statistics presented in this work is based on clinical explanations of death, and a theme of the study is that the reservation was a dangerous place to live during most of the twentieth century because of high death rates resulting from tuberculosis, pneumonia, heart disease, gastrointestinal disorders, and accidents (figure 1.2).

In addition, fetal, infant, and childhood mortality was high among Yakama during the first half of the twentieth century, as large numbers of fetuses, infants, and children under six years of age died (figure 1.3). However, no argument is being made that life on the Yakama Reservation was more dangerous in terms of deaths resulting from disease and accidents than life off the reservation, since no comparative data is available for Plateau Indians living off the reservation in urban or rural settings. As Eugene S. Hunn has stated, the thesis set forth in this study "is strongly indicated by the data," but it has not been proven "that reservations were MORE dangerous places to live for Indian people than off-reservation communities." Hunn is correct, because the comparative data for mortality has not been collected or analyzed for Yakama or other Plateau Indians "who resisted resettlement on the reservation and continued to live about their old village sites."[13] To illuminate the reservation data, comparisons with other populations within the United States are offered, always with an understanding that comparisons are between a small population of Yakama people and much larger populations within the United States.

During much of the twentieth century the Yakama Nation experienced social anomie, depressed over the conditions on the reservation. Recent medical scholarship strongly suggests the relationship of mind and body, emotions and health. Although such Western thought is in its infancy, Native American medicine people, Indian doctors, and spiritual leaders have a general tradition in recognizing the relationship between one's state of mind and one's health.[14] For the Yakama and their neighbors, there can be no doubt that the people were reeling from their recent history with white Americans. In 1855, the United States forced them into a treaty which limited their lands, concentrated several tribes onto a single land base, and destroyed much of their tribal autonomy, freedom, and independence. Between 1855 and 1858, many tribes fought the United States in a military campaign that ended in disaster. Within a matter of a month, soldiers executed several prominent tribal leaders and forced others into exile. After 1859, when the United States ratified the Yakama Treaty, the confederated tribes of the Yakama Nation lived under the thumb of agents, ministers, and pro-government Native American factions. They witnessed Western expansion first-hand as ranchers, farmers, lumber companies, miners, merchants, and other "settlers" overran their former lands. They lost hunting, grazing, fishing, and root grounds. They lost their seasonal rounds by which they obtained their livelihood, and they slipped into a communal depression that weakened their minds and bodies, making them more susceptible to viruses and bacilli.

This is a condition that cannot be quantified or measured scientifically, but anyone—native or non-native—familiar with Native Americans living within the early reservation system will attest to its existence. It surely had some effect on Indian health and one's vulnerability to disease. It is known that Yakama people lived in abject poverty with substandard housing, inadequate food, poor water, few sewer facilities, insufficient health care, little economic opportunity, and limited political power. Everywhere around them people were dying, particularly infants and small children. In addition, large numbers of people between 15 and 29 years of age died of tuberculosis from the 1920s to the 1940s (figure 1.4). This was the Yakama work force, young women and men who made a living so that others might survive. The large number of deaths resulting from tuberculosis and pneumonia (figure 1.5) alone—to say nothing of the high infant mortality rate (figure 1.6) among the Yakama—was sufficient to depress the entire Yakama population. People lived to die and to die young. Still, Yakama people survived and did not vanish from the face of the earth.

No intent is made in this study to "mask" data by hiding statistics that would not support my conclusions. The purpose of the study has been to expose and disclose as much information as possible and, when appropriate, to compare Yakama statistics with data from the *Historical Statistics of the United States: Colonial Times to 1970* and other statistical sources. Scholars interested in discussing aspects of the work are encouraged to correspond with me, so that we might enlarge the discourse about Native American health during the twentieth century. Most often, crude death rates are presented per 100,000 in the population, which is, as one reviewer put it, "the most effective statistical comparison . . . for specific years and diseases/causes, as that helps control for the incomplete reporting for the earlier time periods."[15] Unfortunately, some of the Yakama death rates for the early data are calculated using only a few deaths attributed to a particular cause. Readers must approach this data with caution.

In the case of fetal and infant mortality rates, I provide these comparisons per 1,000 live births. Whenever the national or state statistics were presented in crude death rates per 100,000 in the populations, then the Yakama data is presented in terms of 100,000 in the population. Whenever fetal and infant mortality rates were presented per 1,000 in the population or per 1,000 live births, the Yakama statistics were offered per 1,000 in the population. Crude death rates, fetal death rates, and infant mortality rates are presented in a comparative fashion, in spite of the fact that comparisons are between a small Yakama population with larger populations of the state of Washington and the United States. This is a common scholarly practice, because comparisons are helpful in assessing the importance of rates of death resulting from selected causes among various populations. In addition, as Dr. H. De Lien and J. Nixon Hadley concluded in 1952, "all discussions of Indian health statistics must carry a warning of the dangers involved in interpretation from such a small number of cases."

In comparison to other American populations, the Yakama population was small and the number of cases in any particular year is limited. However, "the use of data consolidated for several years can compensate for this."[16] This study offers comparisons over several years and for particular years as well as some moving averages over time to present a clearer picture of mortality trends during the twentieth century. Comparisons are also helpful in considering issues of gender and age as they relate to death. The work is intended to open the discussion about the relative importance of certain causes of death within the Yakama population and other Native American populations. Future work with the Yakama censuses from 1885 to 1930 will enable scholars to create population pyramids and compare the Yakama population over time with other populations in the world.[17]

According Hunn, the history of Native Americans on "the Columbia Plateau has been first and foremost a history of the ravages of disease . . . which drastically reduced aboriginal populations and disrupted the social and spiritual fabric of Indian life." Hunn argues that "After the treaties were signed and Indians confined to reservations, the significance of introduced diseases faded and political events affecting Indian life took center stage."[18] Indians on the Columbia Plateau had suffered greatly from contagious diseases brought by Europeans, but during the early twentieth century, they were no longer devastated by smallpox, malaria, measles, and fevers. Still, they were affected by contagious diseases such as tuberculosis, pneumonia, gastrointestinal disorders, and influenza. All of these diseases were influenced by the conditions under which the Yakama were forced to live on the reservation, and they all contributed to the general anomie of the people—the social disorganization and cultural destruction of the Yakama. Still, as Hunn, Jeff Zucker, Kay Hummel, Bob Hogfoss, and other scholars have pointed out, once the effects of European diseases played out on the Columbia Plateau, the population began to recover and grow. This was true for the Yakama, just as it was true for Native Americans throughout the United States after 1928, but the twentieth century was marked with new epidemics and a social decline relating to the reservation system.[19]

Members of the Yakama Nation survived, in large part, because of the strength of their spiritual beliefs. In spite of military and political conquest by the United States, and in spite of health and economic collapse, Yakama people maintained their population and witnessed a growth of the population after 1930 (figure 1.7). In 1900, the native population on the Yakama Reservation included 2,309 people, and the population grew slowly until 1920 to 2,910 people. The population remained relatively constant during the 1920s with slight growth and then loss. In 1930, the Yakama population census recorded 2,908 people, two people less than the census a decade before. However, after 1930, the Yakama population began to grow steadily to 3,411 people in 1940 and 3,961 in 1950. In 1960, the Yakama population marked a total of 4,844 men, women, and children, and by 1980, it reached 6,856 people.[20] The maintenance and growth of the Yakama population was due to a high rate of birth after 1930 when the birthrate per 1,000 live births was 19 (Figure 1.8). Between 1935 and 1955, the Yakama birthrate averaged about 28 per 1,000 live births, but in 1960 and 1964, the Yakama birthrate rose to 42 per 1,000 live births (figure 1.9). The Yakama population grew because of rising birthrates as well as the influx onto the reservation of Indians who had been living elsewhere. The general population also grew during the twentieth century because of better public and medical health care, the decline of tuberculosis as the primary killer, improved housing, education, sanitation, and economic opportunities for members of the Yakama Nation on and off the reservation. In any case, while the Yakama people and the Nation as a whole struggled with death on their reservation during the twentieth century, overall the population survived and increased in total numbers.[21]

I chose to focus on the Yakama Reservation because of my interest in the various tribes of the Columbia Plateau who presently reside on this reservation. Furthermore, the study of death on this reservation developed because of the numerous and rich documents relating to death—totaling 3,899—which were collected and preserved by the Yakama Agency (figure 1.1, 1.10). In an appropriations bill in 1884, Congress mandated that the Office of Indian Affairs instruct Indian agencies to collect vital statistics on births and deaths. The government formalized the request on 4 July 1884 in an appropriations act, 23 Statute 76 which required the Office of Indian Affairs to keep vital statistics on Native Americans living on reservations. Thus, collecting and preserving vital statistics of American Indians became a federal matter of the Interior Department, not a territorial or state issue under national law.[22]

However, agents at the Yakama Agency did not create death registers until 1888, although in a few cases the notation "dead" appears beside names in Yakama Tribal censuses prior to that year. In 1888, Commissioner of Indian Affairs John DeWitt complained in his annual report that conducting censuses and collecting vital statistics on the reservation were taxing for agents. He maintained that recording vital statistics was extra labor for agency personnel and required hiring census takers and interpreters. He also complained that the task was made difficult since Indians lived in large geographical areas with few roads where most of the population was mobile. Some of these observations were correct in characterizing the Yakama Reservation, but agents on this reservation made virtually no effort to comply with federal law.[23] Between 1888 and 1907, the Yakama Agency kept only a few death records. These scanty records indicate that the Yakama suffered a total of 9 deaths during the 19 years between 1888 and 1907, which, of course, is a gross under-counting of deaths on the reservation. Only a few deaths were recorded because of inadequate record keeping on the part of the Yakama Agency.

Recording and preserving vital statistics on the Yakama Reservation improved slowly in the first two decades of the twentieth century, particularly after Washington state became a death-registry state. In 1907, officials in Washington state began collecting vital statistics about death, and the Yakama Agency could have kept copies of these Death Certificates created by the state, but they did not do so to any extent until the 1920s (figure 1.1, 1.0). Generally, Death Certificates originated from medical doctors, funeral parlor directors, Indian agents, county coroners, police, and family members. They filed the Death Certificates with the Yakima County Health Department which sent the documents to the Washington State Department of Health. Yakama agents were in a position to facilitate this process and had been charged to do so. However, Yakama agents did not keep many copies of Death Certificates or register their own vital statistics regarding death until the 1920s, and they did so because of national pressure. Kirsten Holm, research specialist for the Washington Center for Health Statistics suggested that the increased number of Death Certificates for Yakama Indians after 1924 was "heavily influenced by outside pressure." That outside pressure was the national Indian reform movement sweeping the country, and it significantly affected death registration of the Yakama population.[24]

Yakama Death Certificates are a significant source of historical information, and this study utilizes those Death Certificates pertaining to Indians on the Yakama Reservation. I used only copies of documents kept by the Yakama Agency, and these documents alone provided me with numerous cases.[25] I have not attempted to sort all Death Certificates for the state of Washington registered after 1907 to determine which of these documents related to Native Americans living on the Yakama Reservation. I have not used this source to track Indian deaths off the reservation, Indian families who were supposed to have moved to the Yakama Reservation in accordance with the treaty of 1855, but who filed patents on lands under the Indian Homestead Act. It would be a monumental task to identify these families, identify individuals within the families, and discover their Death

Certificates—assuming one had been filed. Such a project would take years, and it would have little bearing on a study of Native American deaths on the Yakama Reservation. Thus, this is not a study of death among the non-reservation native population. Besides, during the course of the twentieth century, Indians on the Columbia Plateau lost all their homesteads, and many of these Indian families left their homesteads and moved to the Yakama Reservation. Some of them died on the reservation and are included in the Yakama Death Certificates.

By the 1960s, nearly all Indians that had filed homesteads had been forced off their land and moved to one of the Northwestern reservations to live or had moved to an urban area to work. One scholar has suggested that the Yakama Death Certificates identify 80 percent of the death population on the reservation as full-bloods because many mixed-bloods filed homesteads.[26] This was not the case, and few Yakama filed Indian homestead claims, because their traditional homes were often, but not always, included as part of the reservation. Most Indians who filed home-steads were Palouse, Wenatchee, Klickitat, and various Upper Chinookan-speaking people of the middle Columbia River. Native Americans that filed homesteads were generally full-blood Indians, although they may have been of mixed Indian blood (e.g., Palouse and Wanapum). These people were included in the study if they moved to the Yakama Reservation. Still, the purpose of the work was to study mortality on the Yakama Reservation, not among Indian populations living elsewhere.

Some scholars may be critical of the use of the Death Certificates as the primary data source of this study. The Yakama death records are a solid source—and the best dealing with death—for they provide an unusual insight into Yakama social history. The Death Certificates are far more valuable than the *Annual Reports of the Commissioner of Indian Affairs*, for they provide many more variables, they are more specific, and much more complete. The issue of using Death Certificates over other sources reminds me of a point made by Gary Nash, former President of the Organization of American Historians and Professor Emeritus of History at the University of California, Los Angeles. He once commented that the study of history was much like fishing. If an historian fished in one area, the person landed sources and conclusions that informed in one way. If another historian fished in another body of water, that person might land sources entirely

different. The sources might lead the scholars to different inter-
pretations and conclusions. And so it is with historical inquiry
and the development of historiography.

I have chosen to fish in a sea of nearly 4,000 Death Certificates and have presented my findings in this volume that focuses
primarily on these sources. Yakama Death Certificates have
never been used before to study the fourteen different tribes and
bands on the reservation, and therefore these findings are new.
Unfortunately, few historical studies of Native Americans in
North America have employed Death Certificates, although
Frederick Hoxie of the Newberry Library has done so recently in
his work on the Crow Reservation. In addition to Death Certificates, I have also collected birth registers for the Yakama. The
data base I have created for the Yakama Indian Reservation
provides insights relating to such variables as cause of death, year
of death, age, sex, place of death, and blood quantum. In addition, I have used the 42 years of census data available for the
Yakama Reservation to calculate the number of people living on
the reservation from 1885 to 1931.[27] The censuses are voluminous, but they are not helpful in terms of deaths on the reservation. Some of the early censuses provide short notations if a
person died, but they are not numerous and do not offer such
variables as cause of death, place, age, or other sources of information. The best historical source on death are the Death Certificates, but a future analysis of the census data will offer a
greater understanding of the Yakama population over time.

Although limited use of the Yakama censuses is made for
Death Stalks the Yakama, the Yakama censuses from 1890 to 1930
are currently being coded at ten-year intervals for two separate
projects. The first is to study Yakama families, heads of house-
holds, family sizes, and other matters pertaining to Yakama
families. The second study will utilize census data to study
individuals within the Yakama population, and this will provide
a tremendous data base that will reveal much about the Yakama
population over time. This data will afford an opportunity to
recreate the Yakama population and offer population pyramids
in terms of the young, old, fertility, etc.[28] It will permit a
comparison of the death data with the census data and allow a
rare historical look at one native population, including life tables
to determine the number of people of each sex and of each age
during the era from 1890 to 1930.[29] This data will be compared

to that of the United States population as well as other populations of the world. All of this work is yet to be done, but the present work represents the beginning of an historical process that offers an analysis of death among one Native American population in the early twentieth century.

The present work is divided into five parts, including this short introduction. Readers are asked to consider them as separate elements that are inter-related in a circular fashion, rather than in a linear one. The parts are elements of a plot similar to those found in traditional American Indian stories where the connections between the parts may not appear immediately apparent, but require thought, reflection, and interpretation by those hoping to receive the account's meaning. The presentation of this work is a reflection of the Yakama Reservation itself in as much as there were two reservations or two reservation cultures coexisting at the same time, one native and one white. The reservation is a creation of whites, not Indians, and whites administered the reservation, generating thousands of pages of paper and numerous "laws" by which they governed Indians. White officials of federal, state, and county governments created censuses, Death Certificates, and Birth Registers. The assumptions of their culture are apparent in these documents and others that inform us about life and death on the reservation. At the same time, Native Americans living and dying on the Yakama Reservation represented another culture that the dominant society considered foreign and often contradictory to that of whites. Most glaring are differences in beliefs about religion and causes of death. Indians living on the Yakama Reservation believed that the underlying cause of some deaths was witchcraft, spirit sickness, and rattlesnake medicine, but not once did a recording official attribute an Indian death to one of these causes.

The differing views of causes of death are best illustrated by those surrounding the death of Humishuma, the famous Colville Indian author commonly known as Mourning Dove. The Indian author became ill at the home of Dean and Geraldine Guie in Yakima, Washington, after she divulged that her spirit power was a feather that flowed through her blood stream.[30] Having communicated the nature of her power, in violation of traditional tribal law, Mourning Dove became ill. The Guies summoned medical assistance, but the doctor could not help Mourning Dove. The Guies took Mourning Dove to live with her family on the Colville Reservation, but her condition worsened until 30 July 1936 when she was committed to the state mental hospital at Medical Lake, Washington. On 8 August 1936, Mourning Dove died at the age of 49 of "exhaustion from manic depressive psychosis."[31] In 1988, the author had a conversation with Mary Nelson, a tribal elder from the Colville Reservation. When asked if she had known Mourning Dove, Nelson pointed and shook a finger, saying: "Oh Humishuma, Humishuma! You know what they say! The old people say, Humishuma, she told too much, too much."[32] Medical officials at the state mental hospital recorded that Mourning Dove died of exhaustion, but tribal elders argue that she died of spirit sickness brought on by her transgression of tribal law. She shared too much information, became ill, and died as a result.[33]

The study attempts not to privilege one reservation culture over the other, and therefore, part two of the work introduces Plateau Indian beliefs about death, spirits, and mourning. Part two presents some background material on Yakama people and their neighbors. Particular emphasis is given to the people prior to the reservation system, with information relating to oral literature, diet, spiritual beliefs, faiths, funerals, and burials. This part of the book is not intended to be a definitive discussion of Yakama culture as it relates to death but an introduction to the people and their belief systems. Much of this section is written in the past tense, because this is an historical work, but much of what has been cast in the past tense could have been written in the present tense. Many of the cultural ideas, theories, rituals, ceremonies, and procedures described are alive today and very much a part of the lives of those who follow the ways of the *Wáshat* religion. Readers should never forget that the Yakama enjoy a living, dynamic culture that has changed over time but retained a good deal of its spirit. The third part of the volume presents an introduction to one aspect of white culture on the Yakama Reservation through a discussion of the death data, the non-Indian origin of sources, variables analyzed, and research methodology. Strengths and weaknesses of the statistical data are presented in this section of the work. The fourth part of the book is an analysis of the data. Finally, I provide a short conclusion of the contributions of the study to Native American history in general and Yakama history in particular. I also briefly discuss changes in Yakama Indian health and compare causes of death in the early twentieth century with those of the 1990s. I hope that scholars, public health officials, and tribal people will find the work useful and enlightening. I also hope that the study will encourage other scholars to use Death Certificates to better understand the course of American Indian history in the twentieth century.

Notes

1. Yakama Death Certificates, Yakama Indian Agency Papers, National Archives, Pacific Northwest Region, Seattle, Washington, Record Group 75, hereafter cited as Yakama Death Certificates, NA, PNWR, RG 75. Note that in 1994 the tribe officially changed its name from Yakima to Yakama. When dealing with the tribe and native people living on the reservation, the word Yakama will be used throughout. However, in speaking of the river, county, and city, Yakima will be used.

2. Abdel R. Omran, "Epidemiologic Transition in the United States: The Health Factor in Population Change," *Population Bulletin* 32 (1977): 1.

3. Ibid.

4. Ibid., 4.

5. Ibid., 9.

6. For the most thorough scholarly treatment of disease in the Pacific Northwest in the late eighteenth and early nineteenth centuries, see Robert Thomas Boyd, "The Introduction of Infectious Diseases Among the Indians of the Pacific Northwest, 1774-1874" (Ph.D. dissertation, University of Washington, 1985).

7. *Annual Report of the Commissioner of Indian Affairs, 1900* (Washington, D.C.: Government Printing Office, 1900), 400.

8. Thomas McKeown, "Food, Infection, and Population," *Journal of Interdisciplinary History* 14 (1983): 227. See also Thomas McKeown, *The Modern Rise of Population* (New York: Academic Press, 1976).

9. Ann G. Carmichael, "Infection, Hidden Hunger, and History," *Journal of Interdisciplinary History* 14 (1983): 249.

10. Susan Cotts Watkins and Etienne van de Walle, "Nutrition, Mortality, and Population Size: Malthus' Court of Last Resort," *Journal of Interdisciplinary History* 14 (1983): 218.

11. Ibid., 1-42; Barry M. Popkin, "Nutritional Patterns and Transitions," *Population and Development Review* (1993): 138-57.

12. Samuel H. Preston and Michael R. Haines, *Fatal Years: Child Mortality in Late Nineteenth-Century America* (Princeton: Princeton University Press, 1991), xviii.

13. Eugene S. Hunn to Clifford E. Trafzer, 18 May 1994, author's collection.

14. See the interviews with Candace Pert on "The Chemical Communicators," Margaret Kemeny on "Emotions and the Immune System," David Felten on "The Brain and the Immune System," and Robert Ader, "Conditioned Responses" in Bill Moyers, ed., *Healing and the Mind* (New York: Doubleday, 1993), 177-248.

15. Ibid.

16. H. De Lien and J. Nixon Hadley, "How to Recognize an Indian Health Problem," *Human Organization* (1952): 33.

17. Yakima Census, 1885-1930, NA, PNWR, RG 75.

18. Eugene S. Hunn with James Selam and Family, *Nch'i-Wana, "Big River": Mid-Columbia Indians and Their Land* (Seattle: University of Washington Press, 1990), 32. See also, Jeff Zucker, Kay Hummel, and Bob Hogfoss, *Oregon Indians: Culture, History, and Current Affairs, An Atlas and Introduction* (Portland: Oregon Historical Society, 1983), 152.

19. Russell Thornton, *American Indian Holocaust and Survival: A Population History Since 1492* (Norman: University of Oklahoma Press, 1987), 171-81; C.M. Snipp, *American Indians: The First of This Land* (New York: Russell Sage Foundation, 1989).

20. Yakama Census, 1885-1930, NA, PNWR, RG 75.

21. Henry S. Shryock, Jacob S. Siegel, and Associates, with condensed edition by Edward G. Stockwell, *The Methods and Materials of Demography* (San Diego: Academic Press, 1976), 211-18. Hereafter cited as Shryock, *The Methods and Materials of Demography*.

22. Oral communication, author with Lee Francis, Bureau of Indian Affairs, Washington, D. C., 3 April 1994.

23. *Annual Report of the Commissioner of Indian Affairs, 1888*, xxxiii.

24. Oral communication, author with Kirsten Holm, Center for Health Statistics, Department of Health, Olympia, Washington, 3 April 1994.

25. Yakama Death Certificates, NA, PNWR, RG 75.

26. Reader's Report, "Death Stalks the Yakama," 3 November 1993.

27. Yakama Census, 1885–1930, NA, PNWR, RG 75.

28. Shryock, *The Methods and Materials of Demography*, 107, 134–36, 141–42, 168.

29. Ibid., 262–64.

30. Oral interview by Richard D. Scheuerman with Geraldine Guie, Yakima, Washington, 1983.

31. Jay Miller, ed., *Mourning Dove: A Salishan Autobiography* (Lincoln: University of Nebraska Press, 1990), xxvi. An obituary of Mourning Dove is found in the *Spokesman Review*, 13 August 1936.

32. Oral interview by Clifford E. Trafzer with Mary Nelson, Olympia, Washington, 1988.

33. Several other examples of spirit sickness can be found in the Papers of Lucullus Virgil McWhorter, Manuscripts, Archives, and Special Collections, Holland Library, Washington State University, Pullman, Washington. Hereafter cited as McWhorter Collection, WSU. Used with the permission of the family. See the accounts of Anawhoa (Black Bear), Ikeepsswah (Sitting Rock or Wasco Jim), and others. All of this information is culturally sensitive and should be used in context to Yakama culture since spiritual beliefs surrounding death are central to an understanding of traditional culture.

PART TWO

THE YAKAMA

From Lake Keeschelus in the Cascade Mountains of west central Washington state flows a magnificent river. It snakes its way southeasterly through evergreen forests and into an open, rolling valley. The river cuts across a portion of the Great Columbia Plateau and receives the water of dozens of tributaries such as the Naches, Ahtanum, Toppenish, Satus, and Selah. After a lengthy journey through high ridges, rolling hills, and dark canyons, the river flows into the Columbia River. Since the beginning of time, the Yakima River has been the home of hundreds of Native Americans who share the name of the river and the country.[1] Yakama people lived in this region of the present state of Washington long before the arrival of whites. They lived in a traditional fashion that tied them to the plants and animals, the mountains and the rivers. As one observer has stated: "Their land was their religion, and their religion was the land."[2]

The relationship of the Yakama to the earth, animals, and plants was far more than economic. It was a spiritual relationship that originated at the beginning of time.[3] This axiom is at the heart of Yakama tradition, culture, and history, and without an appreciation of the significance of the earth and spiritual

23

beliefs, there is little understanding of any aspect of Yakama history. This is certainly true of the Yakama beliefs about death, dying, spirits, souls, afterlife, mourning, ceremonials, burials, and memorials. Various aspects of native religion changed with white contact, particularly the form of the traditional faith. However, the basic beliefs of Plateau Indian religion, particularly their relationship with the earth, plants, and animals—the animate and inanimate elements of the spirit world—have remained unchanged through time.

When the earth was young, *Spilyay* (Coyote), the plant people, and the animal people put the world into motion. The ancient stories of the Yakama and other Indians of the Great Columbia Plateau describe earth in transition, a time before humans when the plants and animals made ready for the arrival of humans. According to Andrew George, a Palouse holy man who once lived on the Yakama Reservation, "at the creation, Coyote was present, the symbol of power—teacher of balance, the creator of confusion." Coyote was both creator and destroyer. Indeed, in one ancient story of the Yakama, Coyote outwitted the Five *Tah-Tah Kleah* monsters at the mouth of the Columbia River, destroying a dam created by the monsters and leading the salmon upstream to various tribes of the Inland Northwest.[4] Coyote also helped bring fire to earth by shooting arrows skyward onto a star, creating a ladder used by Beaver to steal fire from living beings from another world.[5] Through his positive actions, Coyote taught the people, and through his negative actions, he did so as well. In fact, his actions were often destructive and confusing, reflecting life itself. Thus, Coyote is a main figure in Yakama spiritual beliefs since he teaches through both his creative and destructive actions. Coyote was also responsible for losing immortality.[6]

According to Yakama tradition, the "law" was established at the time of creation that there would be life and death on earth. At first, Coyote agreed with the law but after several of his family members and friends died, Coyote wanted no more death. So Coyote asked the Creator who lived in the Sky Above to release the people and let them come back to life on earth. Coyote traveled across five great mountains to the west until he reached the Creator and made his plea. The Creator took pity on Coyote and placed the souls of Coyote's family and friends in a deerskin medicine bundle. Creator instructed

Coyote not to open the bundle until he had returned to earth, passing through the five mountains. However, before reaching the fifth mountain, Coyote heard all his friends and relatives singing, laughing, and dancing inside the medicine bundle. Coyote could not control his eager anticipation to visit his relatives again, so he opened the bundle before crossing the fifth mountain. The souls of his loved ones flew back to the Creator, and forevermore, Coyote lost immortality for the people. From then on, there would be death.[7] The theme of death is found in other stories because the Yakama realized the fragile relationship between the living and the dead and the implications of this relationship in their own lives.

To the Yakama and other native people of the Columbia Plateau, death is a "law." Death is a natural part of life, one that is woven into the fabric of native culture. It is a subject often discussed and analyzed in traditional stories, since the people believe that death is a topic to be noted and remembered, not hidden and forgotten. The people recognized that death was natural and occurred all around them. Each year, the spring brought the birth of plants and animals, living things that grew and developed in the spring and summer. Some of the plants and animals died in the fall and winter, only to be reborn in the spring. This was the cycle of life so familiar to the Yakama who lived by traveling in a seasonal round. In the spring of each year the Yakama gathered roots and killed game, and in the early summer, they harvested salmon and gathered more roots and berries. In the fall, they fished, hunted, and gathered as they prepared for winter. At every turn the Yakama killed to survive, bringing death to plants and animals. They did this knowingly, conscious of their actions through thoughts, prayers, and songs. Many of their ceremonies were first food celebrations where they gave thanks to the plants and animals for dying that the people might live. They gave thanks to roots, berries, game, and fish, singing praise to the creation and asking for a renewal of life, a continuum of survival. Death was part of life. This was the law and one which all Yakama understood throughout their lives.

The Yakama lived in accordance with the four seasons of the year, taking life from the earth. In the early spring, they moved to early root grounds. Before the 1750s, they moved on foot, but after this time, they traveled on horses introduced in the

Northwest by Shoshoni from the Rocky Mountains.[8] Each band of Yakama was autonomous, and the members of each decided which root grounds, they would visit. The bands often joined large camps with neighboring tribes. They gathered roots with Cascade, Cayuse, Palouse, Klickitat, Wascos, Wenatchi, Wishram, Wanapum, Walla Walla, and others. They took the nutritious roots in large baskets, baking them in large pits in the ground and drying them in the sun. Women and children did most of this work, securing for their families large quantities of roots to be eaten throughout the year. At these root gatherings, they often raced horses and gambled on the winnings. The encampments offered an opportunity for young people to get to know one another, occasions that led to love and marriage. The people remained at the early root grounds until cliff swallows and mourning doves—mates of salmon people—began their flight inland. With them came the warm Chinook winds and the spring run of salmon.[9]

When word reached the root encampments that salmon had begun to run up the Columbia River, bands dispersed to their own fishing grounds. On family rocks and scaffoldings, men harvested the powerful salmon while women, children, and elders cleaned the fish. The people preserved the salmon by smoking and drying them or by digging huge holes in the river banks and lining them with rocks so that entire salmon could be preserved deep inside the cool earth for use during the upcoming year. The time of the salmon was filled with work, but a good harvest meant plenty of food for months ahead. When the Indians completed their salmon harvest, they gathered roots and berries. They prepared for winter and traveled to visit friends and relatives. In the fall of the year, the people hunted game, gathered late roots, and picked fall berries.[10]

By November, the Yakama had completed the seasonal round, returning to their villages where they awaited the arrival of winter. They spent winters telling stories, delighting in the ancient words of their ancestors. They played string games and devised other forms of entertainment. The people lived in villages that dotted the Yakima River Valley. These ranged in size from fifty to two hundred people, and even more occupied the village of *Cíkik* which was located one mile north of present-day Union Gap. Geographically, the Yakama were divided into two major groups, the Upper Yakama and Lower Yakama.

The Lower Yakama constituted the majority of the people, and they lived in approximately forty-four villages in the lower portion of the Yakima Valley east of the Cascade Mountains. The Upper Yakama had seven villages and were sometimes called the Kittitas, taking the name of the upper valley. They referred to themselves as the *Pswánwapam* or People of the Stony Ground.[11] Eugene S. Hunn pointed out that "There are many folk etymologies of 'yakima.'" Gilbert Smartlowit, a tribal elder from White Swan, told Hunn that the word had its origin as "the pregnant ones" and was part of a traditional story. According to Hunn, "the hills opposite the present city of Yakima were five pregnant women transformed, I believe, by Coyote, during a mythological event." Hunn pointed out that "The term 'yakima' is readily interpreted in Sahaptin: Yak is the verb stem, to be pregnant; -'i' is a nominalizing suffix, i.e., 'one that is pregnant'; and -ma is the plural suffix. It may have originally included a causative prefix 'i-' to make i-yak-i-ma, or those who have been made pregnant. Or, this could all be a post hoc interpretation."[12]

The Yakama were once those Indians who lived in the Yakima River Valley, but they were not isolated in the inland valley, for they traveled extensively on foot and, after the 1750s, by horseback to the Pacific Coast, Rocky Mountains, and Great Plains. They intermarried with people from other regions, and they traveled east to hunt buffalo on the plains of Montana, Idaho, and Wyoming. Contact with other cultures transformed the Yakama who had many neighbors from their surrounding Plateau, a good number of whom were forced onto the Yakama Reservation and are historically incorrectly identified in documents as "Yakama" people. The Yakama adopted the horse and became skilled hunters and fine cavalry fighters. They also appropriated the tipi and used it when they moved temporarily from their permanent homes. Significantly, the Yakama have always been a pragmatic and dynamic people. Perhaps some Yakama met white traders on their travels to Canada or the Pacific Coast, but their first major contact with whites was in 1805 when Meriwether Lewis and William Clark explored the inland Northwest on their way to the Pacific Ocean.[13]

Shortly after Lewis and Clark claimed Yakama land in the name of the United States, the Canadian explorer and trapper,

David Thompson, visited the region and claimed it for Britain. Declarations of ownership to a region by right of discovery were well-known European concepts, but the Yakama had little idea initially of Euro-American intentions in the Northwest. Some Yakama welcomed the opening of trade with the British and Americans, while others scorned the idea, worrying that contact and trade would harm their culture. Although friction existed with some traders, the region became a new market for trade goods. White missionaries—Protestant and Catholic— followed the traders into the area in the 1830s and 1840s, bringing spiritual change to the people. Some Yakama accepted the new teachings, particularly those of the Catholic priests, but others rejected Christianity. Most Yakama practiced their native religion as well as Christianity. Still, all of them were, in some way, influenced by Christianity, and the effects of its presence in their homeland were significant.[14]

Traders brought changes to the Yakama, dividing Indian communities into those who favored trade, those who opposed it, and those who were somewhere in between. The same was true of Christianity which divided Indian people into pro- and anti-Christian groups. Although there had always been tension and division among the people, the introduction of whites into the Yakama country led to new factions over issues, ideas, and items foreign to them. The changes in Yakama culture brought by traders and missionaries were nothing in comparison to changes resulting from white settlers and government policies. The opening of the Oregon Trail in the 1830s and 1840s to the Pacific Coast inaugurated the white invasion of Oregon's Indians and later, Native Americans in Washington Territory, home of the Yakama.[15]

With the immigrants came new governmental institutions that discriminated against Indians. The government of white Americans, historically heralded as democratic, enlightened, and progressive, proved to be dictatorial, oppressive, and regressive, to Native Americans. After establishing a foothold in the Northwest, white immigrants used their governmental institutions to destroy Indian people and their natural title to native lands. By 1853, white power and population in the Northwest were sufficient for the United States to divide Oregon Territory into two large segments—Oregon Territory and Washington Territory. Without their prior permission, knowledge, or participation, the Yakama came under the influence of Isaac Ingalls Stevens who was appointed territorial governor and superintendent of Indian affairs.[16]

In 1854 and 1855, Stevens made a whirlwind treaty tour of the Northwest, attempting to force the tribes of Washington Territory to relinquish title to much of their land, move onto reservations, and accept the domination of the United States. Stevens met with some success in the Puget Sound and on the Coast before turning his attention to the Yakama and other tribes of the Inland Northwest. In May and June of 1855, Stevens held a treaty conference with several Plateau Indian tribes in the Walla Walla Valley. On 9 June, some of the Yakama leaders signed the Yakama Treaty of 1855, in spite of a great controversy that arose over Chief Kamiakin's "touching the pen" and agreeing to sign the document as an act of peace and friendship.[17] Shortly after the treaty council at Walla Walla concluded, white miners discovered gold north of the Spokane River. In the ensuing gold rush, miners trespassed onto Yakama land, stole horses, raped women, killed innocent people, and triggered a war.[18]

When two Yakama men murdered Indian Agent Andrew Jackson Bolon, the United States sent troops into the Yakima Valley. This began a war which lasted intermittently from 1855 to 1858, ending in disastrous consequences for Yakama people. No longer were they free to live and die as their mothers and fathers before them, for they came under the thumb of the United States Army and the Office of Indian Affairs at Fort Simcoe. In addition, during the last campaign conducted by Colonel George Wright, United States soldiers executed a number of tribal leaders, including Owhi and Qualchin, two prominent Yakama chiefs. The blue coats also drove Chief Kamiakin into Canada and Montana. Without the powerful leadership of these important chiefs, the Yakama suffered as a result of American rule. Moreover, the people suffered from depression as they witnessed their ancient patterns of life disappear in a matter of a few years. This was the origin of a societal depression and tribal anomie that was to characterize the people long into the twentieth century, affecting their general health in a negative manner. After 1858, the whites of the United States would direct the lives of Indians, each year assuming more power and determining the fate of the Yakama in terms of physical mobility, foods, housing, family, government, health, and education. After 1858, the United States government determined the course of Yakama people and the consequences of this were devastating.[19]

In 1859, the United States Senate ratified the Yakama Treaty of 1855 by a two-thirds vote and sent it on to the president for his signature.[20] In 1859, the Office of Indian Affairs organized the Yakama Reservation and instituted policies designed to control nearly every aspect of Yakama life. Under Indian agents selected by the government, the Yakama lost much of their ability to determine for themselves their destinies in terms of economics, politics, recreation, social concepts, laws, and religion. Traditionally, Yakama leaders, bands, and families followed the seasonal round, gathering nutritious foods and living in clean, comfortable homes. They looked to Indian doctors—men and women—for preventive information, cures, and advice about pregnancy. With the arrival of non-Indians to the Northwest came new diseases previously unknown to Native Americans—smallpox, measles, and varieties of destructive bacteria and viruses. Many aspects of native culture changed as a result of the white invasion of the Northwest and the takeover of Yakama land by the United States. However, the Yakama did not cave into every demand made by agents, and many held fast to their religious beliefs.[21]

The Office of Indian Affairs forced several different groups of Indians onto the Yakama Reservation. The majority of the Indians were Yakama—Upper and Lower Yakama. However, the reservation also became the home of fourteen tribes and bands, including Wenatchi, Wasco, Wanapum, Tenino, Wishram, Palouse, and others.[22] They were enrolled on the Yakama Reservation and their identity as distinct tribes was lost in birth, marriage, census, and death documents that often identified these native peoples as "Yakama." American Indians living on the Yakama Reservation once spoke several native languages, most prominently Sahaptin, Salish, and Chinook, although today "Sahaptin is the only language still used (with perhaps an occasional rare exception)."[23] Today, the families of these Indians know that they are not technically "Yakama" simply because they live on the Yakama Reservation and are enrolled there. Each family knows their own history and tribal affiliations, and it is common within families to be of mixed Indian heritage. However, agents working for the Office of Indian Affairs usually did not distinguish between the various groups and did not record a person's correct tribe when reporting various documents, including births, deaths, and censuses. Thus, many Indians were placed on the Yakama Reservation where they were lumped together by white agents who generally called them by the generic tribal designation, "Yakama."[24]

By the last half of the nineteenth century, these "Yakama" people had been defeated militarily, but they had not lost their culture. Indeed, the Yakama were not a doomed people destined for extinction. They were not to be counted among the rolls of the "Vanished Americans," for the Yakama survived invasion, conquest, and subjugation. They survived in spite of the reservation system, the strong measures of Indian agents, and American Indian policies designed to "civilize" them and make them over into the white man's Indian. Nevertheless, Yakama life changed as a result of the reservation, particularly in terms of general health. This, of course, is a theory because little data exists regarding the general health of Yakama people prior to white contact and prior to the reservation system. However, this study will show that a large number of Yakama died during the reservation period of the twentieth century, especially infants and children under six years of age. In comparison to the population of Washington state, whites in the United States, and "non-whites" nationally, the Yakama experienced high crude death rates. What is remarkable is that the Yakama population survived in the late nineteenth and early twentieth centuries. In large part, they survived because of their strong spiritual beliefs that dated from the beginning of time. The Yakama proved to be one of the most conservative Indian peoples in terms of belief systems, for they held tenaciously to their traditional religion, in spite of the fact that it was altered and formalized as a result of white contact.[25]

The Washani, Funerals, and Burials

Many Plateau Indians, including Yakama, describe their aboriginal religion as the *Washani* or faith. Contemporary people often refer to their present religion as *Wáshat*. During the 1930s, anthropologist Leslie Spier labeled some of the traditional spiritual beliefs the Guardian Spirit Complex, and this terminology is common in the literature but not on the reservation.[26] In general, there were various aspects of this spiritual belief. Individuals were expected to share their food, wealth, knowledge, and grief. They were expected to live a good life and not harm others. Men and women were to remain free of witchcraft and those who worked their power in a negative manner. Periodically, believers were to purify themselves through the sweat lodge, a small, domed dwelling known to Yakama as *xwyáyc*. Believers sprinkled water over heated stones and prayed while they were inside the sacred dwelling. They sang five series of songs at a time, and many people would sweat for five days in a row. The sweat lodge remains an integral part of traditional Indian religion, and it links humans with the earth and spirits, affording an opening in life through which the spirits can enjoin humans and influence their lives. The sweat lodge purifies people spiritually and offers new or renewed skills, a keen mind, and superior body strength. Traditional Yakama also believe that the sweat lodge experience can cure illnesses—mental, physical, and spiritual. It can also bring luck to a person involved in love or games of chance, two areas of life with similar consequences.[27]

Another element of the old Washani faith is the *wátsa* or vision quest which was undertaken by boys and girls alike so that they could receive their *tah*. Children retreated to secluded spots—often in the mountains—chosen by their families where they fasted for one or more days, usually three to five. During the ordeal, the child was frequently visited by a tutelary spirit or spirits that gave the child power and taught him or her many things. The *tah* taught children a *wánpsa*, or special song, that brought the power to them whenever they needed it. Children also learned the use of special symbols, the way in which to blow whistles, and which power items to carry on their person, such as bundles, feathers, fur, or plants.[28]

Children also learned to avoid certain behavior and to emulate other behavior. The *tah* might teach children to wear certain clothing, paint the body in a particular fashion, or specify the exact time in which they were to do so. The *tah* taught children to dance a special and individual way and instructed them how to use their *tah* power. Children received a variety of powers, including those from such tutelary agents as fog, thunder, clouds, rain, water, birds, bears, insects, trees, moss, and other plants, animals, and features in nature. The power imparted to the children might make them prophets, midwives, chiefs, psychics, psychologists, teachers, hunters, lovers, gamblers, or morticians. Thus, a person's ability to do certain tasks was due to the direction and power received from the *tah*.[29]

One had no choice in the power that would come, since this was decided by spirits on another level of being. When children received a power, they often did not understand it and could not interpret the meaning of the vision. For example, Kamiakin, an important Yakama chief of the mid-nineteenth century, had his vision quest on the snowy slopes of Mount Rainier. His *tah* came to him in the form of a buffalo, and he received his power from the great animal. However, Kamiakin did not understand his power or the meaning of his future life. His mother, Kamoshnite, and father, Tsiyiyak, paid a *twati* or medicine man to spend time with the boy to help him interpret his power. Generally, the Yakama refer to this as bringing out one's power. Kamiakin took a sweat bath with more than one male elder, and they told him that he had a power that would enable him to be a great leader.[30]

Kamiakin, they said, would lead the people on a significant path, a just and right road, but one that would be destructive for the future leader. Nevertheless, they urged Kamiakin to follow the course of action he thought was correct, in spite of criticism. Kamiakin's *tah* helped him become a great leader, one of the most important on the Great Columbia Plateau. He gained power as a warrior and buffalo hunter, in both cases distinguishing himself as a member of the "warrior class" and "buffalo-hunting class." As he became older, he grew in strength and power. When he was approximately twenty-five, he married Sunkhaye, his first cousin and the daughter of Chief Teias. He married his next four wives from among the competing leadership family of Chief Tenax, and by the 1850s, Kamiakin had extended his leadership power among many diverse tribes and bands who recognized him as a powerful leader, but not a "head chief." The latter term was an invention of white Americans, not the Yakama. Kamiakin's life was one of great controversy, as he led his band against the treaty of 1855 and in favor of war against the United States from 1855 to

1858. On his deathbed, he told his family that he had always seen things before they happened, that his *tah* had given him this power. He died a poor man at Rock Lake in the heart of the Palouse country of Washington in 1877 and was buried by his family in the land of his father's people.

Kamiakin's son, Yannaneck, by Sunkhaye, was born in the 1830s and was old enough in the 1850s to fight as a warrior in the Yakama War. As a boy of ten or eleven, Yannaneck had a vision quest at an old hunting camp. In previous years, hunters had killed deer at this site and roasted the meat, making a camp for some time at the place. Deer bones were scattered throughout the abandoned camp, and this was the place that young Yannaneck waited for his *tah*. During one of his nights at the hunting camp, "a terrific electric storm came up" and the night was filled "with a great wind, pouring rain, and beating hail." While Yannaneck sat out the storm in a brush shelter, a voice called to him:

> You do as I tell you and I will give you my power.
> You see that I am old and all weather-checked,
> but this hail does not enter me nor hurt me.
> I resist the beating hail stones which beat upon me
> without harm. Do as I tell you and with my power,
> although the bullets of the enemy strike you like
> a hail storm, you will not be harmed.

Yannaneck learned a special song and received his instructions on how and when to use his deer-bone power. During the Yakama War, he was with a group of warriors surrounded by blue coat soldiers. Young Yannaneck explained that "his body was immune to the arrows and bullets of the enemy" so he would ride for help. He called on his *tah*, sang his sacred song, "then dashed out on his horse, receiving without injury the concentrated fire of the enemy." According to oral tradition, "His clothing was riddled by bullets, not one of which penetrated his body."[31]

The most important power that could be transferred from the spirits to a male or female was the *tamanwas* power, the ability to heal and cure illnesses. A person who received this power was called a *twati* and was far more important within his or her own community than war, civil, or any other type of

leader. Medicine people had both positive power to cure someone, and conversely, negative power to harm others. On one
occasion the author visited a native elder in the hospital at
Toppenish on the Yakama Reservation who was frightened at
the thought that the author would later visit a *twati* they both
knew. Having entered the hospital without first consulting the
traditional holy man, the patient feared that the *twati* would
learn of her action and perhaps turn the power and do the
patient harm, but this did not happen and the patient recovered. Still, it illustrates the fact that contemporary Indians
living on the Yakama Reservation fear the negative power of
Indian doctors and medicine people who can work their power
in a positive and negative fashion.[32]

In general, Yakama agents did not like or trust the *twati,*
and they attempted to extinguish the power of medicine men
and women on the reservation. In the nineteenth century,
Agent James Wilbur worked diligently to stamp out the power
of Indian doctors. In the twentieth century, Agent Donald M.
Carr continued this campaign. The Office of Indian Affairs also
supported the suppression of Indian doctors, instructing Carr
that "you shall do whatever you can to prevent the practice." It
is not surprising that, in 1917, Carr wrote, "It is my belief that
the Indian doctors do a great deal of harm and while the orders
are that no persons shall practice as such, the fact is the Indians
alone can do more to stop the practice than anyone else." Carr
felt that the Indian medicine people "do a great deal of harm,
some of the Indians keep on calling them [Indian doctors] every
time someone gets sick, all of which is wrong." Agents argued
that the medicine men on the reservation "are killing many
young people." Carr instructed his field representatives to
"arrest and try Indian doctors," but his efforts were in vain,
since the Yakama continued to use Indian doctors or suffer
from their negative use of power. In addition to the *twati,* Carr
was also opposed to the Indian Shaker Church which emphasized healing in its ceremonies. Carr argued that "when the[y]
dance, the[y] close the door and all that sweat, spit, and dust
from the floor" was harmful to the participants. He called for a
ban of the Shakers, but he was no more successful in ending the
ceremonies of the Indian Shaker Church than he was in ending
the influence and practices of Indian doctors.[33] Regardless of
the beliefs of the agents and whites associated with the Yakama

Reservation, the *twatis* remained in a central position on the reservation and continued to influence the course of Indian history throughout the first half of the twentieth century.

The Yakama *twati* received their extraordinary power during their vision quests, when the power was transferred to them. Sometimes the power children received was so strong, it struck them down and made them ill. The child received spirit sickness, and it could only be cured with the help of one who had strong spiritual powers. For example, Texanap was a Plateau Indian of mixed Yakama and Wenatchi blood. Her father was a medicine man, and one fall day, he ordered her to return to their former encampment to get his rope. This was an excuse to force Texanap to travel by herself to seek a vision. During the night, she returned to their camp in the mountains to find a horsehair rope he claimed he had left at that place. There, by a pond filled with water bugs, Texanap received her power. The water bugs sang to her and transferred the power. The water helped in the endeavor. The girl lost her ability to walk, because she was afflicted with "spirit sickness." She could not function until her father and other *twati* brought out her power during an all–night ceremony.[34]

To rid Texanap of the spirit sickness, her elders held a ceremony in which they placed a sturdy pole in the middle of a clearing and in a circle set five fires ablaze. The people sang while Texanap's family placed her on a stretcher and carried her to the post. As a community, the people met to bring out her power and cure her spirit sickness. Texanap lay there until she had enough strength to sit up. With the aid of the pole, she struggled to pull herself slowly to her feet. The singing continued long into the night as Texanap gradually regained her ability to stand and walk. In this way, the negative element of the power left her. When she had mastered her legs once again and could keep her balance, she walked over to each of the five fires and placed her face above the burning logs. Then she tossed her head down, allowing her long, black hair to topple over her head into the fire. Her hair did not burn, and she remained above the fire for some time before moving on to each of the five fires. Every time, at each fire, she repeated her actions.

The songs and fires, along with prayers prescribed by her spirit powers, made Texanap a *twati* in her own right. Not only had her elders brought out her spirit sickness, but they had helped her in the personal transformation. This transformation was one in which Texanap was healed of her spirit sickness and at the same time became a healer. In time, she fully received her healing power. From the night of the ceremony forward, Texanap became a *twati* herself, healing people of illnesses and helping others bring out their spirit sicknesses. With the power of water, water bugs, songs, rituals, and five fires, Texanap spent her life working for the betterment of people within the native communities of the central Columbia Plateau. According to Ida Nason, Texanap never charged anyone for her services, travel, board, or lodging. She accepted only that which others wanted to share with her, a tradition followed by most *twati* on the Columbia Plateau, including those, past and present, living on the Yakama Reservation.[35]

As seen in the example above, the gaining of power was not without consequences. The Yakama believed that children must be knowledgeable about receiving power from the spirits both before and after vision quests. Children who did not receive proper instruction from their elders and a trained *twati* could become ill with spirit sickness and never recover. They could have uncontrollable visions or hear voices. If the spirit sickness went untreated, the child could die. Families needed the expertise of a skilled *twati* to bring out spirit sickness and cure people afflicted with problems. The *twati* had intimate knowledge of sickness and knew exactly how to counteract the ill effects of the spirit sickness. Traditionally, spirit sickness was a significant and dangerous cause of death among Yakama people. However, medicine doctors knew how to bring out the sickness and destroy its negative power. They also knew how to handle cases involving witchcraft.[36]

In addition to spirit sickness, Yakama believed that children and adults were vulnerable to the intentional misuse of power by medicine people, men and women who could turn their positive power into destructive, even deadly power. This was another explanation of death among traditional Yakama, but one which could be countered by trained Indian doctors. When witchcraft occurred, the person exorcising the evil power was a *twati* and the witch was referred to as a *watayíylam*. Helen Schuster, a renowned scholar who has studied the Yakama for years, reported that one person told her about witchcraft.

If someone witches a person, Indian doctor will say, "I'm
gonna get it out, it's easy." Then he'll say in Indian, "*Áwnaš alp
ákusa; áwnaš áwunpsa . . .*" "I'm gonna get 'em." Then if he do
that right, then maybe you'll hear that that witch die, pass
away in three days.[37]

Parents feared witchcraft being worked against them and
their children. If parents did not follow society's rules, the
negative power could be turned against them and their children.
A member of the family could become ill and die if he or she
walked on a sacred site, killed an animal ignoring a prescribed
ritual, looked at a sacred totem, or exchanged cross words with
a *twati*. In addition, people could become ill and die as a result
of other cultural transgressions, and their children could also
suffer as a result. After the arrival of non-Indians, some
Yakama attributed the large number of deaths of infants and
children to the misdeeds of their parents. The deadly power of
a *twati* was (and is) sometimes labeled witchcraft and viewed as
a misuse of power. However, witchcraft stemmed from an
individual, not an organized group of people who lived solely
to do harm to others.[38]

In 1924, Evan W. Estep, agent of the Yakama Reservation,
wrote to the Commissioner of Indian Affairs to complain that
the Indians under his charge still believed in the power of
medicine people, in spite of the efforts of Christian missionaries among the people. "I had presumed," Estep wrote, "that the
Yakimas were far enough advanced in civilization to be pretty
well rid of the medicine man influence but longer acquaintance
with them shows that the superstition with them is just as great
as with the less advanced tribes." He also commented that "the
Yakimas are cursed not only with medicine men but with
medicine women." Agent Estep was surprised to learn that
nearly "all of the Indians believe in the ability of this select
fraternity who throw 'spells,' and 'spirits' over the sick."

Even the Yakama leadership believed in the misuse of power
by medicine people, including Chief Meninick who reported to
the agent that "the medicine fraternity had threatened him."
The chief pointed out to the agent that "something should be
done and called attention to the fact that more deaths had

occurred during the present year than was usually the case and that the medicine men were bragging about their ability to kill." While Chief Meninick took seriously the threats against him by traditional medicine people, the agent did not believe in the power of the *twati* to harm and kill people. And not once did a death record kept at the Yakama Agency report that a person had died as a result of the power of medicine people. This was typical of whites in authority at the agency, but Yakama people certainly believed in such powers and many still do.[39]

Along with witchcraft and spirit sickness, Yakama also believed that rattlesnake power was a major cause of death. A person with this power was not necessarily a witch or *twati*, although witches and medicine people had the ability to work their power against others through rattlesnake power.[40] The person with rattlesnake power sent an invisible spirit of a rattlesnake into someone's home, automobile, path, or workplace. When the snake had an opportunity, it struck the victim, placing its poisonous spirit power into the body. People who were attacked by rattlesnake power had to be treated by a *twati* immediately who could counteract the poison of the spirit snake, locate the invisible rattler, kill it, and remove the spirit from the body and premises. When the *twati* removed the rattlesnake spirit power from the person's body, that person got well, since the *twati* had greater power than the rattlesnake person or the rattlesnake spirit. However, if the child or adult went untreated, the rattlesnake power killed the individual.[41]

Yakama views of diseases were important elements of Yakama culture, and they changed with the introduction of diseases brought by white Europeans and Americans. Prior to white contact, spirit sickness, witchcraft, and rattlesnake power were underlying explanations of death within Plateau Indian communities, and they were Native American in origin. The new diseases brought by whites devastated Indian populations in the eighteenth and nineteenth centuries, physically and spiritually destroying native peoples. Still, Yakama people believed in the power of traditional Indian medicine, positive and negative, but such native beliefs did not fit neatly into the Western way of viewing disease, accidents, and death. Historically, non-Indians on the reservation recorded that deaths among children, for example, were due to automobile accidents, tuberculosis, pneumonia, or premature birth, but a Yakama might argue that the best explanation of some deaths were spirit sickness, witchcraft, or rattlesnake power that was not dealt with properly. Hunn stated that these violent and purposive "*explanations* of deaths were (and to some extent still are) widely believed to be the ultimate cause of many deaths, but I don't know that we can say they were considered the cause of *most* deaths at that time."[42] Such beliefs by Yakama were rarely—if ever—taken seriously by Indian agents on the Yakama Reservation. These native explanations of death never appeared as causes of death in documents created by whites.

In addition to spiritual disorders, Yakama died of physical problems resulting from accidents, old age, infections, war, and the like. They called the discomfort of disease *páyuwi,* and in some cases they had medicine or *tawtnúk* with which to treat the physical ailment.[43] Hunn and his native teacher, James Selam, have identified over seventy-five medicinal plants that the Yakama and their neighbors used for healing. Elders had the knowledge to heal through medicinal plants, and this knowledge was general and shared by many people. Medicinal plants were used to treat people suffering from fever, colds, diarrhea, blood disorders, headaches, stomach ailments, rheumatism, influenza, spider bites, venereal disease, infection, tuberculosis, pneumonia, worms, coughs, arthritis, trench mouth, and a host of other physical problems. Thus, the Yakama used medicinal plants to treat physical problems and disease introduced by whites. However, the Yakama did not have specialized herbologists who treated such disorders in response to "white man's disease," but rather they continued to rely on common knowledge employed by elders within families.[44]

Significantly, the Yakama often believed that the root cause of physical problems was spiritual in nature. Prior to white contact, the Yakama may have been exposed to some diseases, but they did not suffer from epidemics of smallpox, measles, influenza, malaria, whooping cough, and pneumonia. When whites introduced diseases to the Yakama, Indian doctors attempted to heal the people of the scourges with the knowledge available to them. Thus, Yakama doctors were general practitioners, holy people, pharmacists, shamans, and psychologists, and they recognized no division between mind and body. Indian doctors and Yakama people suffered several epidemics before the introduction of the reservation system, but they were largely powerless to prevent the waves of death that swept across the Columbia Plateau in the nineteenth century and those that struck the native population in the twentieth century. The result, initially, was the depopulation of the Yakama and other native people of the Northwest before their recovery in the twentieth century.

Smallpox was the first disease to strike Northwestern Indians. The first epidemic probably started in 1775, the result of sailors from trading vessels off the Northwest coast introducing it to native peoples.[45] Another smallpox epidemic traveled up the Missouri River in 1783, but its effect on the Plateau is unknown. In 1801, still another smallpox epidemic spread among the native people of the Northwest, "reducing the original population to about one half by the time of Lewis and Clark's" expedition in 1805. In 1824–25, and in 1853, smallpox likely killed more Indians. In 1830, "fever and ague" broke out at Fort Vancouver, infecting native people for four years. The epidemic may well have been malaria, although it was linked to an outbreak of influenza, and the "mortality directly or indirectly attributable to this scourge . . . is 90%!" The malaria outbreak in 1830 reportedly "did not spread much above The Dalles," and Plateau Indians probably died instead from influenza, although the number of deaths is not known.[46] In 1844, scarlet fever and whooping cough spread across the Columbia Plateau, and scarlet fever struck again in 1846. In 1847, measles moved across the Plateau, taking the lives of many Indians and sparking the killings of Marcus and Narcissa Whitman and others at the Whitman Mission which, in turn, triggered the Cayuse Indian War of 1848.[47] These epidemics and the new diseases that followed killed numerous Yakama and their neighbors. Diseases depopulated the native peoples and strained the social, cultural, and spiritual fabric of Yakama society whose *twati* could not undo the horrors of white diseases.

During the era under examination from 1888 to 1964, recording agents never listed the primary or secondary causes of death as spirit sickness, rattlesnake power, or witchcraft. Furthermore, never once did they suggest that the cause of death of a person living on the Yakama Reservation might be due to his or her violating social or cultural beliefs.[48] Yet the Yakama believed that one might become dangerously ill or die if he or she transgressed the moral norm, insulted a medicine person, or committed an infraction against a sacred place, item, or tradition. All of this was outside the world of white officials working for the territory, state, county, or Office of Indian Affairs, but it was very much a part of Yakama culture. Indeed, such Indian ideas were not part of the Western system of thought regarding explanations of death, but they certainly were and are an important element of Yakama culture that must be kept in mind when discussing death among Yakama Indians. Spirit sickness and other aspects of positive and negative spirit power are still significant components of Yakama culture and ones that must be understood in terms of the Yakama perspective of death.[49]

Death and rebirth are other elements of the Washani religion, and historically, there have been many Native Americans from the Columbia Plateau who died and were reborn in order to communicate with the Creator and return to the earth with a message from the Supreme Power. This is an important element of the Washani faith and one that fits well into the traditional belief system of Yakama and other Native Americans. The Yakama had long believed in the power of dreams and visions, including spirit travels to learn from plant, animal, mist, and other spirits. Indeed, children received their power in this way, and they carried this force with them into adulthood. Therefore, when holy men and women explained that they had died, traveled to another world, and returned with new power, this experience fit well into Yakama belief systems.[50] Whites living during the nineteenth century scoffed at such ideas, perhaps forgetting the visions and spirit helpers received by Daniel, Jesus, and Paul.[51] Whites often poked fun at native beliefs, calling the holy people fakes, frauds, wizards, and witches.[52] Regardless of their assessment of the Yakama and other Indian prophets, it is imperative to realize that the Indians believed in the holy people and their afterlife experiences. This belief by the Yakama changed their traditional religion, adding form, doctrine, and ritual to the rich Washani past.

There were numerous Indian prophets from the Northwest who influenced the Yakama. Some of them include Luls of the Umatilla, Toohoolhoolzote of the Nez Perce, Husishusis Kute of the Palouse, and Smohalla of the Wanapum. There is no question that Smohalla had a tremendous influence on nearly

all Indians living on the Columbia Plateau during the nineteenth century, but he was not alone in his afterlife experiences. Among the Yakama, Kotiahkan was the most important
prophet who died and was reborn. He was from Union Gap and
was the son of Chief Showaway, brother of Chief Kamiakin.
Kotiahkan had approximately three hundred followers, and
according to traditional accounts, he had received his power
when he died and traveled to the other world where the creative force taught him the Dance of the Dead.[53]

He learned many things from the spirit people, and he was
sent back to earth to teach others. Kotiahkan, like many Indian
prophets, taught the people to *washat* or dance in a stylized
fashion which required the participant to jump up and down
while standing in a circle with others, move counterclockwise
to the beat of a drum, and sing songs taught to the prophet by
the spirits.[54] He taught that the spirits lived in the land of the
dead, where they would remain until returning to the earth one
day. He taught them ritual and doctrine, new songs and ceremony to be performed each Sunday in the longhouse.
Kotiahkan performed a religious ritual with the help of seven
drums and a congregation that used feathered fans held in the
right hand when worshipping. Men stood on one side of the
longhouse while women worshipped on the other side.
Together the prophet and congregation sent their prayers and
praises to their creator, *Saghalee Tyee* (Our Father), *Nami Piap*
(Elder Brother), or *Honyawat* (Creator).[55]

Changes that occurred in the Washani religion came about,
in part, as a result of white contact and coincided with the
invasion of Yakama lands by white traders, missionaries,
soldiers, and politicians. In addition, disease and death came
with whites, and the bacilli and viruses introduced to Native
Americans on the Columbia Plateau created a new climate for
religious change. Epidemics of smallpox, influenza, and measles
killed hundreds of Northwestern Indians, and to combat the
scourges, Indians turned to their most respected holy people
who prayed for divine help. In 1934, Cora DuBois learned from
an Indian living on the Warm Springs Reservation in Oregon
that "One man died" and returned to earth where he informed
the people that he had spoken with the Creator who "told him
to have this Indian religion every seven days and sing." According to this Yakama person, the prophet received the message "a

long time back when people were dying like flies." There were many prophets from many parts of the Northwest, and nearly all of them received similar messages in like fashion, learning similar songs, rituals, and doctrines.[56]

Prophets like Kotiahkan and others added new dimensions to the traditional Washani religion that were influenced, in part, by Christianity. In the pre-contact era, the Yakama reportedly had no belief in "heaven," a place where the spirit of the dead traveled after death. However, traditional stories refer to souls living in another world, a world visited by Coyote and others. Although the Yakama had communal services to celebrate a thanksgiving of such sacred foods as roots, berries, and salmon, they usually did not meet communally to worship except for mid-winter ceremonies. The Yakama congregated for *wánpsa* or winter sings, but this was only done in the winter from December through March, and the activity was not held weekly. After the arrival of missionaries, many prophets gathered their followers to worship every Sunday. They met as a congregation in the longhouse to sing, dance, and pray in accordance with the messages received by the holy people of the faith.[57]

Washani prophets often returned from their afterlife experiences with messages from the Almighty regarding worship, songs, dances, and beliefs. Although Washani worshipers prayed for good health, the Washani faith did not center around healing, since curing was an element of the old culture assigned to Indian elders and doctors. While the Washani did not focus on curing, the Indian Shaker Church and Feather religion did center around curing—and both continue to do so today. Jake Hunt, a Klickitat Indian from the village of Husum on White Salmon River, was the most important early prophet of the Feather religion, which was known to many Indians as the *Waptashi*. With the power of eagle feathers and mirrors, believers in the Feather religion became healers. This came to be an established religion on many Northwestern reservations, and it is a belief system that is still practiced today. Like the Waptashi, the Indian Shaker Church also has elements of healing as part of its doctrine. In 1892, John Slocum, a Nisqually Indian from Mud Bay, Washington, established the Indian Shaker Church. Like other prophets, Slocum died and was resurrected, returning to earth with a new religion. The most important component of the Shake was healing through the power of the Holy Spirit. "When people are sick," Slocum once stated, "we pray to God to cure us. We pray that he take the evil away and leave the good."[58]

Some Indians living on the Yakama Reservation followed the new ways of Christianity, Waptashi, or Shake. Others remained within the fold of the Washani faith and traditional Indian doctors but would periodically call on the leaders of the other religions if they needed help in curing a loved one. The Yakama used white medical doctors, if the physicians of the Indian Office or United States Army were nearby. When a physician or nurse matron of the Indian health division was available, most Yakama sought their advice and help in medical matters. Unfortunately, Congress did not make a federal appropriation specifically for American Indian health until 1911, and designated funds for Indian health were not provided every year. The medical element of the Office of Indian Affairs targeted tuberculosis and health education, but the funding was limited. In 1920, Congress mandated that a senior administrator from the Public Health Service work with the Indian Office to advise the agency about health issues. In 1921, Congress passed the Snyder Act which appropriated special funds for Indian health and "resulted in the creation of the Bureau of Indian Affairs Health Division and the appointment of district medical directors." The Public Health Services aided the Indian Bureau in terms of health after 1926, and in 1954, Congress transferred the responsibility of Indian health to the Public Health Service in the Department of Health, Education, and Welfare—known today as Health and Human Services. All of these developments affected Yakama people.

If a clinic or hospital was located in their area, the Indians traveled to these medical institutions for aid. But while pursuing this line of foreign aid, the people also sought the help of *twati* and use of traditional cures, including the sweat lodge, to solve their medical problems. Often Yakama families used a variety of medical services, Indian and non-Indian, to cure their people. Sometimes these various techniques of curing worked, but at other times people died. In the 1870s and 1880s, the Yakama Agency received some support from the Indian Medical Services of the Indian Office but most often the Yakama received medical care from the Army at Fort Simcoe.

In the 1890s, the Indian Office dispatched nurses and field matrons to the Indians in an attempt to educate people about hygiene. Between 1915 and 1917, Yakama Agent Donald M. Carr employed a few field matrons to educate mothers about the care of their babies and families. Esther M. Sprague ran this program, but Carr complained that he did not have sufficient funds to educate the people about disease prevention, nor could he hospitalize the sick because he had no hospital.[59] Indeed, the Office of Indian Affairs did not build a hospital on the reservation until 1928, and the Indian Office never built a sanitarium for tuberculosis patients on the Yakama Reservation. Instead, Indians from the Yakama Reservation were most often transferred to the Nez Perce Reservation in Idaho.[60]

Death

In the human experience, perhaps nothing is more emotional for people than death. Not only do humans contemplate their own death, but they consider the death of friends and loved ones. This is particularly true of parents and grandparents when they consider the protection, care, and cure of their children. The Yakama Indians were and are no different, since they enjoyed a strong family structure for their immediate and extended families. They also were tied to one another through their longhouses and churches. When a child became ill, Yakama parents and grandparents sought the medical care of traditional *twati* and elders (particularly women) with medicinal knowledge. They also sought the help of white doctors and nurses at hospitals and clinics, provided these people and facilities were available.[61] However, one of the impediments for Yakama people in receiving medical care was transportation.

Poor transportation systems on the Yakama Reservation during much of the twentieth century influenced the health and life of native peoples living on the reservation because they could not easily travel to health facilities. During much of the twentieth century, Yakama families used horses and wagons for travel, and if they had an automobile or pickup truck, it was generally a used vehicle and not always reliable. Moreover, roads on the Yakama Reservation developed from foot paths, horse trails, and wagon roads. Some of these were hazardous, particularly after Yakama people began using pickup trucks and automobiles. The roads were of a poor quality, hampering transportation to and from medical personnel at Fort Simcoe or Toppenish. In addition, until the latter portion of the twentieth century, most Yakama families did not have telephones and could not call for help. Thus, medical attention was difficult to obtain because of transportation and communication problems.[62]

Still, Yakama families did their best to protect and cure their children and other members of their families. There were times when traditional medicine or that of white people healed the person. Other times patients grew sick and died. This was an important moment in the lives of Yakama people. As one person put it: "When somebody die, that's when our religion really goes strong."

Sometimes family members received warnings that illnesses, accidents, or deaths were about to occur. Animals such as coyotes and ravens tell people about impending deaths. Owls also carried messages at times, landing near people and "speaking" to them of death or disaster. According to Hunn, "the call of the owl is interpreted in Sahaptin as: pá-tkwatan-a [has eaten] tanínshin [arrowhead + subject suffix] X; 'Arrowhead [I believe, a symbol of death] has eaten X,' . . . with X the name of the victim. The owl doesn't always clearly call out the victim's name, in which case it is 'just calling.'"[63] One person saw a great horned owl *(patkwatana)* two nights in a row, warning that death or illness was near. The man's wife became ill after the second night and went into shock. She nearly died of dehydration and had to be hospitalized. "The owl was in a tree outside my home," the man reported, "and after calling me it flew right at me and turned sharply. It was there for two nights."[64] The woman lived through the experience, but the owl had warned that a death–threatening event was imminent.

Like many Indians, the Yakama believe that animals can carry a message of problems ahead and death. Ghosts or *cis* also can give warnings that danger lies ahead. Ghosts might exhibit their baleful deeds by tapping on windows, beds, or doors, thereby announcing that they are present and plan to do some harm to the living. They may also tell a Yakama that someone is about to lose the *hawluk* which is described as a vapor of continuously changing form, the life force or breath that is different from the soul. When people lose their *hawluk*, they also lose the *wsqiswit*, which has no literal translation in English but is also like one's life or soul.[65]

When a person died, the *hawluk* and *wsquiswit* left the body. The onslaught of death brought danger to the family from maleficent ghosts. The ghosts could contaminate the surviving members of the family, and the family either used the sweat lodge for five consecutive days or washed in water containing the purifying effects of wild rose bush. Members of a family also attached wild rose bushes on their doors and walls to protect them from ghosts. These techniques normally warded off ghosts, although the Yakama continually worried about the ill effects of ghosts. Furthermore, the family ended its use of the deceased's name for a minimum of one year after which the family underwent a memorial service for the one who had died. When a member of a Yakama family died, the family could not eat meat or fish because to do so would delay the metamorphosis of the body from flesh into earth. The Yakama believed that seven days after burial, the skin of the deceased became earth. If members of the family did not follow the food restrictions, the dead person's transformation would be delayed and the living would develop "dead skin" on their own bodies. In the past, when a person died, the body was taken to the home or longhouse for preparation. Today, the body is taken to a mortuary where it is prepared before being transported home for a traditional service.[66]

If the deceased and family did not desire a traditional Washani burial, then the family had the person's body handled at a mortuary and services held at a church. However, the body of one who was a member of the longhouse was washed and dressed in traditional buckskin by a relative of the same sex who also adorned the deceased person's hair with small eagle feathers and animal fur. An in-law of the dead often made a buckskin outfit for the deceased, including moccasins. If the deceased was a man, usually his sister-in-law placed a bone breastplate onto his chest and an eagle feather fan into his hands. When a woman died, she was dressed in a buckskin dress. As the funeral preparations were being made, guests arrived at the house. People from many parts of the country, but especially from Northwestern reservations, attended the funeral. They brought food and gifts for the family of the deceased, and they offered money to help pay expenses.[67]

The body was prepared on the day of death. During the next three days and nights, followers of the Washani held a mourning ceremony which began in the home of the deceased and was moved for the next two days and nights to the longhouse. Worshipers placed the body of the deceased in a casket, and when it was moved to the longhouse, they placed it on a tule mat situated on top of a platform. Plants and flowers decorated the area around the body which was laid in state in an east–west direction with the head toward the west, the direction of death and afterlife. When the deceased was female, mourners usually draped three colorful Pendleton shawls over the casket, and when the deceased was male, they put three Pendleton blankets over it. Family members placed favorite personal items of the dead on the shawls or blankets, draping the coffin, including knitting needles, spools of thread, fishing equipment shotguns, beadwork, quilts, deer rifles, and drums. While preparing the body for the funeral, people combed the hair of the deceased, and the person's hair was carefully taken from the comb and kept in a small bag that the mourners placed on the platform near the coffin. In addition, mourners wrapped a few dishes in a white cloth, placing the bundle in the southwest corner of the platform. The family used these dishes during the service to symbolically feed the dead person.[68]

For three nights, mourners sang, danced, prayed, keened, and cried. On the third night, they held the final and largest ceremony. This was the night before burial, and most mourners had arrived from other Northwestern locations. Wearing buckskin clothing and moccasins, mourners sat on the floor for a large feast provided and served by the friends and family of the deceased. Before the dinner, drums began to beat, and people assembled around the inside of the longhouse. A bell ringer called people to prayer, holding a brass school bell in his hand and ringing it above his head in proper time. The people followed an old ritual, blessing the water, salmon, roots, and berries. They ate foods in communion, each time blessing the gifts of creation. While the family and guests ate, an in-law "fed" the deceased using the bundle of dishes left on the platform near the coffin. When mourners finished the meal, the bell ringer rang the bell, and the people stood facing east, singing a Wáshat song. They ended with the traditional "AYYYYYYY" before turning countersunwise in place and sitting down. Females cleared the food from the area, while males gathered and washed dishes.[69]

While men and women removed food and dishes, a male drum leader and seven drummers began a series of seven sacred songs of the Wáshat. After a small rest, the drummers continued with two new series of seven songs each. As the men drummed and sang, women and children danced in place in a hopping motion. After the third series of songs, the leader invited mourners to speak their hearts about the deceased.[70] Helen Schuster reported that, at one funeral, a mourner stepped forward to share these words:

> We follow our Indian way and try to do good for one another. That's no written law. We're all brothers. So we all help one another. I hear white mens gonna start studying our Indian way, learn how to live together instead of all that turmoil.[71]

The singing continued until roughly 2 AM when mourners provided coffee and sandwiches for everyone. The singing ended for an hour, so that the singers and assembled crowd could have a break. When mourners finished their snacks, drummers offered another set of seven songs. People prayed, sang, danced, talked, and slept until the first light of morning. Then mourners washed, combed their hair, and prepared for breakfast. This was the morning of the fifth day, the day of the burial. Following the breakfast feast, people cleared food and dishes, cleaning the area before beginning the burial phase of the Wáshat ceremony. Generally around 10 AM, drummers began a series of seven songs. As mourners sang, they first faced toward the center of the longhouse, then east, west, and east.[72]

The first set of seven songs was followed by another set of the same number, before people began moving counterclockwise around the longhouse and past the coffin to view the deceased for the last time. While most mourners filed out of the Longhouse to organize the funeral procession, friends and family of the deceased wrapped the Pendleton blankets or shawls around the body. They also placed the associated grave goods into the casket, including the bag of hair taken from the comb used on the person who had died. These same people carried the coffin to the hearse, which in the past was a wagon and today is a pickup truck or an automobile. Traditionally, mourners followed the body to the cemetery on foot or on horseback, but today they travel in cars and pickup trucks. Immediately behind the hearse is a pickup truck with seats in the back. Bell ringers sit in these seats as well as seven women mourners who keen on the way to the cemetery. The pickup is followed by automobiles and trucks, all of which follow the hearse to the cemetery.[73]

Before the early twentieth century, the Yakama and their neighbors usually wrapped the body in tule mats and placed it in crevices of hills and mountains. They also buried their dead in designated cemeteries, where they interred a number of people from the same area, village, or family. These cemeteries were and are sacred places to Yakama who revere the remains of their loved ones—long past and recent past. They respect the dead of their own people as well as the dead of other nations, believing that it was and is sacrilege to disturb burials of any people. Many believe that the spirits of the dead cannot rest if their bones are taken out of the earth or generally disturbed by contractors, pot hunters, etc. When the United States began building power dams in the Pacific Northwest, construction crews ruined several burials in canyons along inland rivers, including Snake River. Sometimes archaeologists working for the federal government raided Indian burials to preserve choice specimens for university collections before water from a new dam inundated the locations.

Mary Jim, a Palouse elder living today on the Yakama Reservation, still laments the theft of her grandfather from the family's cemetery on an island in Snake River. She remembers the night in the 1960s when an amphibious vehicle came up Snake River and moved onto the island. While white men dug up the grave, Mary's cousin, Charlie Jim, paddled out to chase the whites away. "They took our grandpa," Mary Jim reported years later, "they took him. They went across. And they took that grave. They dug a hole and we hollered at them. Charlie Jim went out to tell them to stop. We waved red flags at them, telling them, stop. Then the car went through the water and on the ground too. We didn't know how to chase them or where they went. And we reported this to the agency, but they never helped us."[74] Unfortunately, the Palouse were not able to prevent the "scholars" from stealing the canoe coffin that contained the remains of Mary and Charlie's grandfather.[75]

It was not uncommon for Plateau people to bury their dead in large, cedar canoes that were usually cut from side to side in the middle of the canoe. The body was placed in one side of the canoe, while the other side of the canoe was inverted and placed on top of the bottom half. It served as a lid and covered the body, thus forming a canoe coffin. This was the type of canoe coffin in which Fishhook Jim, Mary and Charlie Jim's grandfather, had been interred. Then the Indians placed the canoe coffin deep into the ground with appropriate grave goods that often became the treasures of museums and private collections. During the twentieth century, such traditional burial practices ended on the reservation, where the Office of Indian Affairs and Christian missionaries urged people to adopt new funeral practices. However, while some of the form of the funeral has changed, the entire process is native to the region, retaining several elements of traditional ritual, song, and ceremony.

Some Yakama hold a graveside service today, singing Wáshat songs and saying prayers for the deceased and their family. If the coffin is metal, the family might enclose it in a pine or cedar box. In a traditional burial, the people placed unwoven tule rushes in the grave and lowered the casket onto them. Before lowering the coffin into the grave, the Yakama usually brushed the sides and bottom of the grave with wild rose bush in order to protect the site and the body from ghosts. They also placed three woven tule mats onto the coffin, before mourners moved counter-clockwise around the grave singing as they walked around the top of it. Men, women, and children tossed handfuls of dirt into the grave, before several people shoveled dirt onto the coffin. When the grave was covered, mourners usually placed flowers, prayer sticks, prayer feathers, or other objects on the grave to commemorate the dead. If the person had been a bell ringer of the Washani faith, they often placed a brass bell on top of the grave.[76]

When the burial ended, everyone returned to the longhouse to "make tears" and eulogize the dead. Women keened with heads bowed and men cried. Mourners made speeches, speaking what would be their final words for months about the deceased. They used the name of the dead until they put his or her name to rest. It would not be spoken for one year, when the community released the family from mourning. They held a feast, honoring the dead and the family before preparing for a give-away. Traditional give-aways were major events for the family who gave away nearly every material item in their household, keeping only a few items for themselves in remembrance of their loved one. This was to help the family by removing items that would remind them of the one they had lost. Also, by giving away all of their belongings, they did not fight over the estate and were dependent on their extended family and community for help in living through the mourning period. Giveaways also served as a redistribution of wealth; this giving and then receiving served to create strong bonds between family and friends.

In addition to presenting to their friends and relatives all of the items owned by the deceased, the family also gave away Pendleton blankets and shawls, jewelry, beadwork, belts, clothing, appliances, tools, saddles, and the like. These were gifts for those who had helped the family during their personal tragedy. Familial elders of the deceased made a special effort to remember all of the mourners who had helped make funeral arrangements, prepare and clothe the body, cook meals for the services, clean dishes, and arrange for the drummers, dancers, and singers. Within the Yakama community, it was a great honor to give away all of one's possessions, and it was an honor to be remembered by receiving a gift in this fashion. There were many degrees of give-aways during the twentieth century, but it was very common to have some give-away ceremony after the death of a loved one.

However, in the case of the death of one's spouse, Yakama traditionalism employed a complex widower's or widow's trade known as *paláxsiks*.[77] This culturally significant practice was detrimental to the people, for through it, the Yakama transferred infectious baccili from household to household. If the person had died of tuberculosis, pneumonia, gastrointestinal disorders, or another infectious diseases, the bacilli moved with the unsanitized material items thus spreading the infection and killing others. In 1923, Dr. Margaret W. Koenig pointed out these problems in her study, *Tuberculosis Among the Nebraska Winnebago: A Social Study on an Indian Reservation*, indicating that the people spread tuberculosis by using common cups, spoons, dishes, and pipes. The Ho Chunk (Winnebagos) also transmitted the disease through direct expectoration and through "bed clothes seldom changed, aired or washed." Importantly, she noted that upon death, families gave away all these personal items. This was no less true for the Yakama than it was the Ho Chunk and numerous other tribes throughout North America.[78]

Five days after the burial, the family of the deceased Yakama visited their in-law, bringing with them a bundle of black clothes and a black handkerchief for the person to wear in mourning. During the first half of the twentieth century, the family cut the hair of the deceased's spouse and placed the black handkerchief around the person's hair and chin. "Long before my time," reported Mrs. Caesar Williams in 1917, about the 1840s to 1850s, "they rubbed pitch over the face of a widow woman, to which they added a coating of charcoal. The face was covered all over in this way and she had to wear it for five years." In addition to blackening the face to indicate a state of mourning, the Yakama cut the person's hair; "sometimes it was cut almost as close as if it was shaved from the head."[79] If the person had given away their cooking and eating utensils, clothing, blankets, and other necessary items, the family of the deceased replaced them. They helped the spouse and his or her children in this way, placing items on tule mats either inside or outside the house, depending on the time of year. In addition to their involvement in this widower's or widow's give-away, families of the two groups also traded items with each other. This formed a new bond between the two groups, and it honored them both in remembrance of the dead. The spouse and the deceased person's family exchanged traditional items, including roots, berries, fish and game. They traded other foods as well as buckskin clothing, cornhusk bags, blankets, shawls, modern clothing, and other bundles of goods.

During the *paláxsiks*, the two groups shared Wáshat prayers before and after a large dinner. The dead was eulogized without mentioning his or her name, and the two families simply shared some time with each other. They also made it clear to each other that during the forthcoming year, they would be helpful to one another. During this year, the spouse and children were prohibited from participating in any ceremonies until they had completed their mourning process. After mourning for a year, families of the deceased returned to the spouse's home to "release" him or her from mourning. In the past, the family of the deceased brought a person to replace the one who had died, someone the spouse could marry. Although this is not a common practice today, everyone is aware of the tradition, for they speak openly of it.

In 1917, Lucullus V. McWhorter attended a memorial feast "given by a mother in memory of her son who had died two years before." During this observance, the mother supervised "the feast with some ceremony, and spoke in tones of grief and tenderness of her departed son." On another occasion, McWhorter attended the "Parade of the Dead" and a traditional dance celebrating the life of a person who had died some time before. During this memorial gathering, "a man stepped from the crowd of spectators to the head of the dance-space and spoke in low tones to the head man who repeated his message in a loud voice":

> My brother used to dance with you here: but now he is gone. I feel sad. Your work strikes my mind strongly and my heart is filled with sorrow. I donate this two dollars and a half to be distributed among the people.[80]

At the same memorial ceremony attended by McWhorter, "a woman and her daughter stepped from the crowd to the place of the head man near the west end of the dance pavilion constructed of pole-work and brush." The two added "three shawls, one native made basket bag and $3.00 cash." These were given to the people in honor of the daughter whose name was changed that day to *Wal-lec-wauk*. After a number of people gave gifts honoring the living and dead, the head man distributed the gifts to key individuals present that day. One of the gifts, a traditional Yakama hand-woven bag, was presented to Dr. Griffith, the agency doctor who was going to Europe to fight in World War I and who could use the bag "to carry his ammunition, as he was going across the water to fight the Germans." Thus, the memorial service had several functions, including memorials honoring the dead, namings, and redistribution of wealth to honor significant individuals within the Yakama community. The ceremony also served as a communal blessing to all with the intent to protect everyone from misfortune, ill health, and death.[81]

Following the memorial service, the family returned to the spouse's home with new clothing, fresh linens, bright blankets, pots, pans, and other useful items. This was a time when both families formally thanked each other for their many kindnesses and began honoring the deceased with memorial parades which were once conducted on painted horses. They also celebrated with dinners, dances, and give-aways. People were free to speak the name of the dead, share photos of them, and wear their buckskin clothing. Throughout the memorial ceremony, people would call out the name of the dead to honor and remember them. Through words, stories, material items, and ceremonies, the Yakama kept the person alive and in motion, weaving his or her life into the collective memory of the people.[82]

Memorial ceremonies for the dead often took place on such holidays as Washington's Birthday on 22 February, Memorial Day in May, Yakama Nation Encampment on 4 July, Thanksgiving week, and in December before New Year's Eve. Memorial events were related to, but sometimes separate from, the Lament of the Dead, another memorial ceremony. Native Americans of the Columbia Plateau held laments of the dead during root, salmon, and berry feasts. At these events, people gave thanks to the creation for the First Foods ceremonies and came together to remember their loved ones. For example, Mary Jim, helped organize Palouse, Wallula, Wanapum, and other relatives of her people who gather each summer near her traditional home of Tasawicks along the Snake River. As a group, they meet to celebrate their own survival and lament their removal to the reservations, far from the graves of their children, parents, grandparents, and people. They cry together, not out of bitterness for past policies of the United States government, but for their dead, many of whom are buried beneath the waters of man-made lakes where their relatives cannot visit the graves or wrap their bones.[83]

During the nineteenth century and early twentieth century, the Yakama continued an age-old practice of reclothing the dead and adorning the deceased with grave goods. Generally one year after burial, the people unearthed the remains of their loved ones. They cleaned the flesh from the bones and wrapped the remains in animal hides or blankets. Family members sang and prayed, honoring the dead in this fashion. They often continued this process for years in remembrance of the deceased. In 1878, the family of Kamiakin, the famous Yakama-Palouse leader, returned to the chief's grave one year after his burial. The family planned to dig up the remains to clean his bones and wrap them in ritual fashion. When they opened the grave, they found that his burial had been desecrated.

A white rancher who hated Kamiakin had led a scientist to the grave and had helped the "scholar" cut off Kamiakin's head with a shovel. The scientist tore off Kamiakin's head, placed it in a gunny sack, and took it to his lab for analysis. When the family found that Kamiakin's remains had been disturbed, they cleaned the remaining bones and reburied them on lands belonging to a friendly white rancher in eastern Washington Territory. Members of the family knew the location of the grave, and they returned periodically to pray for the spirit of the famous chief. Kamiakin's head has never been recovered, and the associated grave goods buried with him have not been repatriated. However, some members of the Indian and non-Indian communities continue to search for Kamiakin's head so that it can be repatriated and reburied in the heart of the Columbia Plateau. The desecration of his grave is just one example of many that have occurred in the Pacific Northwest.[84]

The Yakama and their neighbors have faced a continual onslaught by ghouls, construction crews, and government agencies that disregard and discredit the spiritual beliefs of Northwestern Indians in reference to their dead. Many Indians believe that when the graves of their ancestors are desecrated, the souls of the dead are also disturbed, unable to rest until they are placed back into the bosom of the earth. Among the Yakama, death was and is a significant part of the life cycle, and their views of death and the causation of death had little to do with the accounting of deaths made by the territory, state, or Office of Indian Affairs. Indeed, the traditional Yakama views of the causation of death are not reflected once in the Death Certificates, but throughout the era from 1888 to 1964, Yakama people continued to believe that their friends and relatives died as a result of traditional causes, as well as disease and circumstances brought by whites to the Yakama Nation.

Notes

1. Eugene S. Hunn has presented an excellent case for the term, Yakama, to be native to the people in Hunn to Trafzer, 18 May 1994. According to Lucullus Virgil McWhorter, the term Yakama stems from a Salish word, *Yah-ah-ka-ma*, which means "a growing family." The Yakama spread out across present-day east central Washington and extended their influence among many different tribes, including Salish-speaking Indians of eastern Washington. The noted anthropologist, Verne Ray, suggests that Yakama means "the pregnant ones," and early trappers working for the North West Company referred to the tribe as Eyakema or Yackamens. The Lower Yakama probably called themselves *Waptailmin* or "Narrow River People," while the Upper Yakama referred to themselves as *Pswánwapum*, "Stony Rock People." See L.V. McWhorter, *Tragedy at Wahk-Shum, Prelude to the Yakima Indian War, 1855-1856* (Fairfield, Washington: Ye Galleon Press, 1968), 45; Verne F. Ray, "Native Villages and Groupings of the Columbia Basin," *Pacific Northwest Quarterly* 27 (1936): 123; Alexander Ross, *The Fur Hunters of the Far West*, edited by Kenneth A. Spaulding (Norman: University of Oklahoma Press, 1956), 22; Ross Cox, *The Columbia River*, edited by Edgar I. and Jane R. Stewart (Norman: University of Oklahoma Press, 1957), 259; Helen Hersh Schuster, "Yakima Indian Traditionalism: A Study in Continuity and Change" (Ph.D. dissertation, University of Washington, 1975), 30-31, 35; George Gibbs, "Report of Mr. George Gibbs to Captain McClellan on the Indian Tribes of the Territory of Washington," 33d Cong., 1st sess., H. Doc. 91, 407; reprinted as *Indian Tribes of Washington Territory* (Fairfield, Washington: Ye Galleon Press, 1972), hereafter cited as *Gibbs' Report*.

2. Document 520A, McWhorter Collection, WSU.

3. Ella Clark, "George Gibbs' Account of Indian Mythology in Oregon and Washington Territories," *Oregon Historical Quarterly* 56 (1955-56): 293-325 and 57 (1955-56): 124-67; Ella Clark, *Indian Legends of the Pacific Northwest* (Berkeley: University of

California Press, 1953); Virginia Beavert, ed., *The Way It Was: Anaku Iwacha* (State of Washington: Franklin Press, 1974); and Clifford E. Trafzer, ed., "Grandmother, Grandfather, and Old Wolf," unpublished manuscript containing sixty-four traditional stories of the Columbia Plateau. The stories contain the spiritual relationship of animal and plant people who prepared the world for the coming of Yakama and other native people of the Northwest.

4. Coyote scolded two of the *Tah Tah Kleah* monsters for eating too many animal people, and in a journey from the Yakama country south toward the Columbia River, two of the sisters died, leaving their remains on the face of the earth. This site is a sacred place to Yakama who go to this place to pray, sing, and make offerings. Andrew George to Clifford E. Trafzer, 29 May 1987, author's collection.

5. Listening Coyote, "How Beaver Stole the Fire," November, 1921, McWhorter Collection, WSU.

6. George to Trafzer, 29 March 1987.

7. Blazing Bush, "How Coyote Lost Immortality," McWhorter Collection, WSU. The story is presented in Nashone, *Grandmother's Stories of the Northwest* (Newcastle, California: Sierra Oaks Publishing Company, 1987), 37-39.

8. Shoshoni Indians introduced the horse to the people of the Northwest, attaining them through trade with various Plains tribes. See Francis Haines, "The Northward Spread of Horses Among the Plains Indians," *American Anthropologist* 40 (1938): 429-37.

9. Verne E. Ray, *Cultural Relations in the Plateau of Northwestern America* (Los Angeles: Southwest Museum, 1939); "Economic Use of the Tribal Territory of the Yakima," United States Claims Commission, Dockets 47 and 47-A, National Archives, RG 279; Hunn, *Nch'i-Wana*, 138-200.

10. Ibid.

11. *Gibbs' Report*, 407.

12. Hunn to Trafzer, 18 May 1994.

13. Helen H. Schuster, *The Yakima* (New York: Chelsea House Publishers, 1990), 43-44; Gary E. Moulton, ed., *The Journals of the*

Lewis and Clark Expedition, 7 vols. (Lincoln: University of Nebraska Press, 1988), 5:271-313; Hunn, *Nch'i-Wana*, 228-68.

14. Clifford E. Trafzer and Richard D. Scheuerman, *Renegade Tribe: The Palouse Indians and the Invasion of the Inland Pacific Northwest* (Pullman: Washington State University Press, 1986), 21-30; Clifford E. Trafzer and Margery Ann Beach, "Smohalla, The Washani, and Religion as a Factor in Northwestern Indian History," *American Indian Quarterly* 9 (1985): 309-24.

15. Dorothy O. Johansen, ed., *Robert Newell's Memoranda* (Portland, Oregon: Champoeg Press, 1959); Phillip A. Rollins, ed., *The Discovery of the Oregon Trail* (New York: Charles Scribner's Sons, 1935).

16. Kent D. Richards, "Isaac I. Stevens and Federal Military Power in Washington Territory," *Pacific Northwest Quarterly* 63 (1972): 81-86; Trafzer and Scheuerman, *Renegade Tribe*, 31.

17. Kent D. Richards, *Isaac I. Stevens: Young Man In A Hurry* (Provo: Brigham Young University Press, 1979), 211-34.

18. For information on the Yakama Treaty, see Documents Relating to Negotiations of Ratified and Unratified Treaties of the United States, National Archives, RG 75, Microfilm T494, Reel 5; Charles S. Kappler, *Indian Affairs, Laws and Treaties*, 2 vols. (Washington, D.C.: Government Printing Office, 1940), 2:698-702; Alvin Josephy, Jr., *The Nez Perce Indians and the Opening of the Northwest* (New Haven: Yale University Press, 1965), 345; William Compton Brown, *The Indian Side of the Story* (Spokane, Washington: C. W. Hill Printing Co., 1961), 131-35; Andrew Jackson Splawn, *Ka-mi-akin, Last Hero of the Yakimas* (Portland, Oregon: Stationary and Printing Co., 1917), 37-41.

19. Trafzer and Scheuerman, *Renegade Tribe*, 60-92.

20. Kappler, *Indian Affairs*, 2: 698-702.

21. Schuster, "Yakima Indian Traditionalism," 486-88.

22. Kappler, *Indian Affairs*, 2: 698-702; Robert H. Ruby and John A. Brown, *A Guide to the Indian Tribes of the Pacific Northwest* (Norman: University of Oklahoma Press, 1986), 58-62.

23. Hunn to Trafzer, 18 May 1994.

24. Ruby and Brown, *A Guide to the Indian Tribes of the Pacific Northwest*, 58-62; oral interview by Clifford E. Trafzer and

Richard D. Scheuerman with Mary Jim, 10 November 1979, Yakima, Washington, author's collection.

25. Jeffrey C. Reichwein, *Emergence of Native American Nationalism in the Columbia Plateau* (New York: Garland Publishing Co., 1990), 323–24; Schuster, "Yakima Indian Traditionalism," 480–82.

26. Leslie Spier, "The Prophet Dance of the Northwest and Its Derivations: The Source of the Ghost Dance," *General Series in Anthropology* (Menasha, Wisconsin: George Banta Publishing Co., 1935).

27. Schuster, "Yakima Indian Traditionalism," 152–53. Although Humishuma (Mourning Dove) was a Salish–speaking Indian from the Colville Reservation, her discussion of "The Sweatlodge Deity" is instructive and similar to that of other Plateau Indians, including the Yakama. Her original presentation is in a manuscript held by Geraldine Guie, Yakima, Washington; see also Jay Miller, ed., *Mourning Dove: A Salishan Autobiography*, 36–38; Schuster, *The Yakima*, 36.

28. Oral interview by Clifford E. Trafzer, Richard Scheuerman, and Lee Ann Smith with Andrew George, Yakama Reservation, 15 November 1980; author's collection; oral interview by Clifford E. Trafzer and Richard D. Scheuerman with Mary Jim, 10 November 1980, Yakama Reservation; Schuster, "Yakima Indian Traditionalism," 114–17.

29. Trafzer and Scheuerman, *Renegade Tribe*, 33; G. B. Kuykendall, "Spirit Beliefs," manuscript, Click Relander Collection, Yakima Valley Regional Library, Yakima, Washington; hereafter cited as Relander Collection.

30. Brown, *The Indian Side of the Story*, 60–80; Splawn, *Ka-mi-akin*, 17–21; Trafzer and Scheuerman, *Renegade Tribe*, 33.

31. Click Relander, "Sophie Williams," Interview in *Colville and Palouse Notes*, 45, Relander Collection; Harry Painter, "New Light on Chief Kamiakin," *Walla Walla Union Bulletin*, 18 March 1945; oral interview by Richard Scheuerman with Emily Peone, January 1981, Colville Reservation, Scheuerman Collection, Endicott, Washington; Roland Huff to William Compton Brown, 29 September 1949, William Compton Brown Collection, Manuscripts, Archives and Special Collections, E. O. Holland Library, Washington State University, Pullman; hereafter cited as Brown Collection, WSU.

32. Schuster, *The Yakima*, 36. The tribal elder mentioned is still alive and has asked not to be identified.

33. Robert Ruby and John Brown, *John Slocum and the Indian Shaker Church* (Norman: University of Oklahoma Press, 1996).

34. Video with Ida Nason, "Everything Change, Everything Change," information regarding her mother, Texanap, Ellensburg Public Library, Ellensburg, Washington.

35. Ibid.

36. Schuster, "Yakima Indian Traditionalism," 159, 163, 167; Robert H. Ruby and John A. Brown, *Dreamer-Prophets of the Columbia Plateau* (Norman: University of Oklahoma Press, 1989), 13.

37. Ibid., 170.

38. Ibid., 168; oral interview by Clifford E. Trafzer and Richard D. Scheuerman with Mary Jim, 10 November 1980, Yakama Reservation.

39. Evan W. Estep to Commissioner of Indian Affairs, 10 October 1924, NA, PNWR, RG 75, File on M. L. V. McWhorter, Seattle.

40. Specific examples of rattlesnake medicine are found in the McWhorter Collection, WSU, some of which are published in Donald M. Hines, *Magic In The Mountains, The Yakima Shaman: Power & Practice* (Issaquah, Washington: Great Eagle Publishing, 1993), 105-27.

41. Schuster, "Yakima Indian Traditionalism," 167, 171. See also the many accounts of rattlesnake medicine in the McWhorter Collection, WSU.

42. Hunn to Trafzer, 18 May 1994; Hunn, *Nch'i-Wana*, 193.

43. Hunn, *Nch'i-Wana*, 193.

44. Ibid., 351-58; Boyd, "The Introduction to Infectious Diseases Among the Indians of the Pacific Northwest, 1774-1874, "145-73.

45. Boyd, "The Introduction of Infectious Diseases Among the Indians of the Pacific Northwest, 1774-1874," 71-128.

46. Ibid.; Hunn, *Nch'i-Wana*, 27-31.

47. Ibid., 31-32, 242.

48. Yakama Death Certificates, NA, PNWR, RG 75.

49. Schuster, "Yakima Indian Traditionalism," 118, 167, 174; Hunn, *Nch'i-Wana*, 236-41; Hunn to Trafzer, 18 May 1994.

50. Ruby and Brown, *Dreamer-Prophets of the Columbia Plateau*, 12-15, 29-37; Trafzer and Beach, "Smohalla, the Washani, and Religion as a Factor in Northwestern Indian History," 73-76; James Mooney, "The Ghost Dance Religion and the Sioux Outbreak of 1890," *Fourteenth Annual Report of the Bureau of American Ethnology* (Washington, D.C.: Government Printing Office, 1896), 723-31; Cora DuBois, "The Feather Cult of the Middle Columbia," *General Series in Anthropology* 7 (Menasha, Wisc.: The George Banta Publishing Co., 1938), 15; Spier, *The Prophet Dance*, 8.

51. The Bible contains numerous stories about spirits, visions, and supernatural events. See *Holy Bible* (New York: Oxford University Press, 1973).

52. A recently published example of the racist and biased views of one white toward Yakama and other Plateau Indians spiritual beliefs is found in an introduction written by a nineteenth-century military doctor named George Kuykendall, in Hines, *Magic In The Mountains*, 23-71.

53. Mooney, *The Ghost Dance Religion*, 723-31; Edward S. Curtis, "The Yakima," *The North American Indians*, 7 (Norwood, Massachusetts: Plimpton Press, 1911), 362; Hunn, *Nch'i-Wana*, 241-57.

54. Mooney, *The Ghost Dance Religion*, 728-30; Spier, *The Prophet Dance*, 8.

55. Andrew George to Clifford E. Trafzer, 29 March 1987, author's collection.

56. DuBois, *The Feather Cult*, 9.

57. Blazing Bush, "How Coyote Lost Immortality," McWhorter Collection, WSU; Schuster, "Yakima Indian Traditionalism," 160.

58. Homer G. Barnett, *Indian Shakers: A Messianic Cult of the Pacific Northwest* (Carbondale: Southern Illinois University Press, 1972), 35-38; Weston La Barre, *Ghost Dance: Origins of Religion* (New York: Dell Publishing Company, 1972), 199; Al Logan Slagle, "Tolowa Indian Shakers and the Role of Prophecy at Smith River, California," *American Indian Prophets*, edited by Clifford E. Trafzer (Newcastle, California: Sierra Oaks Publishing Company,

1986), 115-16. Robert Ruby and John Brown, *John Slocum and the Indian Shaker Church.*"

59. Carr to Commissioner of Indian Affairs, 7 June 1917, and Sprague to Carr, 5 May 1917, "Health & Hospitalization Records and Reports, 1912-1940," Box 264, NA, PNWR, RG 75.

60. Ibid.

61. Schuster, "Yakima Indian Traditionalism," 175-76.+

62. Clifford E. Trafzer, "The Twentieth Century Horse: The Role of the Pickup Truck in Indian Country," *American Indian Identity: Today's Changing Perspectives*, Clifford E. Trafzer, ed. (Newcastle, California: Sierra Oaks Publishing Company, 1989), 27-40.

63. Hunn to Trafzer, 18 May 1994; Hunn, *Nch'i-Wana*, 234.

64. Schuster, "Yakima Indian Traditionalism," 440. The author had a telephone conversation with a person about the owl and agreed not to identify the individual who shared this story in December, 1992. Also see the warning of death that came to James Selam, in Hunn, *Nch'i-Wana*, 232.

65. Schuster, "Yakima Indian Traditionalism," 156-57.

66. Ibid., 139. For an outstanding study of the belief in souls and afterlife experiences, see Ake Hultkrantz, *Conceptions of the Soul Among North American Indians* (Stockholm: The Ethnographic Museum of Sweden, 1953) and *The North American Indian Orpheus Tradition* (Stockholm: The Ethnographical Museum of Sweden, 1957).

67. Schuster, "Yakima Indian Traditionalism," 440-41.

68. Ibid., 441.

69. Ibid., 442.

70. Ibid., 443.

71. Ibid.

72. Oral interview by Clifford E. Trafzer with Richard D. Scheuerman, 19 March 1993, Endicott, Washington.

73. Schuster, "Yakima Indian Traditionalism," 443-44; Craig Lesley of Portland, Oregon, sent a photograph to the author depicting a funeral on Warm Springs Reservation. In the photograph, Andrew George, a prominent Washani leader, is seated in a horse-drawn wagon carrying a casket, ringing a bell while

mourners walk behind the rig. Traditional burials are not uncommon today on Northwestern Indian reservations.

74. Mary Jim, "A Palouse Indian Speaks," *Bunchgrass Historian* 8 (1980): 21-22.

75. Oral interview by Trafzer and Scheuerman with Mary Jim, 10 and 17 November 1979.

76. Ibid.

77. Schuster, "Yakima Indian Traditionalism," 140.

78. Margaret W. Koenig, *Tuberculosis Among the Nebraska Winnebago: A Social Study on an Indian Reservation* (Lincoln: Nebraska State Historical Society, 1921), 33-34.

79. L. V. McWhorter, "Customs of the Yakimas: A Feast and Donation in Memory of the Dead" and "A Feast of Thanksgiving For Recovery From Serious Illness." July 1917, File 1526, McWhorter Collection, WSU.

80. Ibid.

81. Ibid.

82. Ibid.; Schuster, 142.

83. Trafzer and Scheuerman, *Renegade Tribe*, 143.

84. Ibid., 101-2. The author and Richard Scheuerman have spent fifteen years trying to locate Kamiakin's head to have it repatriated.

PART THREE

YAKAMA DEATH CERTIFICATES: THEORETICAL AND METHODOLOGICAL ORIENTATIONS

Death Stalks the Yakama is an outgrowth of work on the history of the Palouse Indians, native people who once lived along the Snake River from roughly west of what is today Clarkston, Washington, to Pasco, Washington. In the process of doing research for *Renegade Tribe: The Palouse Indians and the Invasion of the Inland Pacific Northwest*, several important documents from the Yakama Indian Agency Papers from the National Archives, Pacific Northwest Region, in Seattle were discovered.[1] Archivist Joyce Justice helped locate this material. Yakama Agency documents are important for several reasons. Obviously, they enhance our understanding of Palouse Indians, since they were party to the Yakama Treaty of 1855, and because some Palouse moved onto the Yakama Reservation. In addition, the many volumes of Yakama Indian Agency Letterbooks record outgoing and incoming correspondence by agents, doctors, and educators employed by the agency. But there is also a rich body of documents that required quantitative evaluation. Included in the collection were nearly 4,000 Death Certificates (the early data before 1907 was recorded on Death Registers) recorded by state and county officials (figure 1.1).

Death information contained in these documents was provided at the most fundamental level by family members of the deceased, medical doctors, Indian agents, county coroners, funeral officials, and others. In addition, officials recorded numerous births in registers during the twentieth century; this information proved useful, as well. Copies of these documents originally were kept at the agency and were subsequently preserved in the National Archives, Pacific Northwest Region, in Seattle. All death documents pertaining to the Yakama Reservation were copied, including several duplicates that were sorted and discarded. Yakama death records were available for the years from 1888 to 1964, although the Office of Indian Affairs kept few Death Registers or Certificates until after 1910 (figures 1.1, 1.10). During that time, government agents collected only 29 death records, a gross under-counting of those who actually died.

Before the 1920s, Yakama agents apparently made little effort to obtain copies of documents from state officials responsible for recording deaths on the reservation and they made almost no effort to keep vital statistics on births and deaths as mandated by the federal government in 1884. Although incomplete for the early years, the data for the 1888–1964 period is a rich source of information, providing a unique opportunity to examine the issue of death over time on a single Indian reservation. Little has been published on the reservation era of Yakama and other Plateau Indians in general. Almost nothing has been written that examines death over time on the Yakama Reservation in particular. As a result, the discovery of a cache of Yakama Death Certificates and related material offered an opportunity to examine a poorly understood part of American Indian history.

Furthermore, such a study offers insights into epidemiological transitions among a diverse Yakama population over an extended period.[2] In general, Native Americans have not been studied historically in terms of death over time, and certainly no one had produced an analysis of death among the fourteen different tribes and bands that form the Yakama Nation.[3] Although these Indians included Yakama, Klickitat, Wenatchi, Wanapum, Wasco, Wishram, Palouse, and others, the Death Certificates identified nearly all Indians who lived on the reservation as "Yakama" based purely on their place of residence. As a result, there was no way to identify a person's tribal background or to determine if they were related more to one group than another. Documents simply are not clear on this point. Unfortunately, there was no possibility of comparing and contrasting death statistics relating to each group. And since no similar data set exists from Death Certificates or Registers from another reservation, no comparative examination could be undertaken. However, comparisons are offered between the Yakama population and the general population of the State of Washington, the general white and African American populations in the United States, and other non-white groups in the United States.

As a theoretical framework from which to cast the Yakama death study, the works of Abdel R. Omran and Barry M. Popkin were employed. Omran's work on epidemiological transition led to an analysis of the Yakama data in terms of three overlapping transitional periods: (1) the Age of Pestilence and Famine (ca. 1800–1920s), (2) Age of Receding Pandemics (ca. 1900–1940s), (3) the Age of Degenerative Man–Made Diseases (1940s–present).[4] The era of pre–Euro–American contact, is beyond the scope of this study, but the first period dealt with here began before the arrival of Meriwether Lewis and William Clark in 1805, when Plateau Indians were introduced to European diseases transmitted by sailors and traders transmitted to the Pacific Northwest Coast.[5] The Age of Pestilence and Famine was disastrous for the Yakama and their neighbors, as smallpox, measles, malaria, influenza, fevers, and other contagious diseases ravaged the native population of the region. In addition, tuberculosis, pneumonia, and influenza also spread among Native Americans, indiscriminately killing large numbers of people. By 1900, many of these diseases were in retreat, while others continued and grew in importance as causes of death among the Yakama. During the Age of Receding Pandemics, smallpox, malaria, fever, and measles nearly disappeared as important causes of death, but tuberculosis, pneumonia, and influenza continued to be major causes of death.

Yakama Death Certificates provide enormous insights into these causes of death as the Age of Pestilence merged with the Age of Receding Pandemics during the first few decades of the twentieth century. This was an important era in Yakama history, and it is the central focus of this study. Although the government of the United States created the Yakama Reservation through the Yakama Treaty of 1855, the reservation system among this diverse native population did not blossom until the late 1860s. Under the forceful administration of Methodist minister and agent, "Father" James H. Wilbur the government's policies of "civilizing" and Christianizing the various tribes and bands on the Yakama Reservation emerged.[6] Wilbur and agents who followed him tried to "civilize" the native population on the reservation by urging them to become farmers and ranchers rather than hunters, gatherers, and fishers.

For approximately thirty years, roughly from 1870 to 1900, native people living on the Yakama Reservation witnessed a radical cultural, social, and economic transformation of their native lands as white ranchers, farmers, politicians, bureaucrats, ministers, bankers, road builders, and a host of other whites invaded their country, altering nearly every aspect of traditional Indian life. The process accelerated in the twentieth century as hunting, root, berry, and grazing areas declined or were destroyed. Indians living on the reservation lost their native foods which were closely tied to their spiritual beliefs. They lost more than their economy, for they lost important threads of their social fabric. Indians living on the Yakama Reservation faced a social and cultural calamity by 1900, a communal depression that corresponded with a serious rise of infectious diseases, particularly tubercular infection. Between 1900 and 1940, the Yakama population suffered greatly from tuberculosis, pneumonia, and gastrointestinal disorders, bacterial infections that preyed on a Yakama host seriously injured by government Indian policies and the reservation system.[7]

By the 1940s, the Yakama entered a new era when tuberculosis, gastrointestinal disorders, and pneumonia declined in importance as central causes of death. After World War II, the Yakama entered the Age of Degenerative Man–Made Diseases as heart disease, cancer, and accidents became the primary causes of death on the Yakama Reservation. And during the late twentieth century, alcohol-related deaths, diabetes, murders, and suicides rose significantly as accidental deaths and pneumonia continued to plague Yakama people, just as they had throughout the earlier part of the twentieth century (figures 1.5, 3.1, 3.2, 3.3, 3.4). Barry Popkin has argued that part of this transition to man-made disease is a predictable product of nutrition related to "modernization." He is correct in terms of Yakama people who had lost nearly all of their traditional foods by the 1940s, and after World War II, consumed refined foods which they purchased with cash earned through labor, leases, and family businesses.[8]

The cause and number of deaths, as well as infant and childhood mortality, on the Yakama Reservation are of primary importance in this study. Samuel Preston and Michael Haines have dealt with infant and child mortality by focusing primarily on whites and African Americans.[9] Unfortunately, they were not able to examine data specifically on Native Americans. Their data is suggestive, however, since African Americans and American Indians had lower literacy rates and income than white Americans, and both Native Americans and African Americans had much higher death rates and infant mortality rates during the twentieth century than did whites.[10] Since the present work is based on a native population, it may be of value to demographic historians as well as those interested in Native American history. Yakama Death Certificates may also be of interest to scholars of Native American Studies because they offer an opportunity to test a common axiom of Native American history. Some scholars have argued that once the United States forced Indians onto reservations, a large number of Indians—but most markedly infants and children—died as a result of the reservation system. Unfortunately, accurate data on population, disease, infant mortality, and death rates do not exist for the period prior to the reservation system, so no comparison can be made regarding Yakama deaths prior to 1855 when the United States established the reservation system.[11]

Prior to their contact with whites, the Yakama suffered severe eye ailments and they died from many causes, but few from communicable diseases such as smallpox, measles, typhoid, typhus, tuberculosis, influenza, or pneumonia. Although the Indians of the Columbia Plateau did not live a utopian life before white contact, their standard of living was relatively high due to diet, climate, housing, and availability of resources. Most tribes, even those from other language families, coexisted in relative peace, sharing food resources, geography, and ceremonies. The people generally spoke more than one Indian language and they intermarried with each other, forming familial bonds that exist to this day. According to John R. Weeks, Director of the International Population Center and noted scholar, "prior to European contact mortality rates were high, but were more *predictable.*" He affirms that Yakama people "knew what to expect as causes of death (even if they identified them differently than does the Western medical model). Predictability is, of course, a staple of human existence."[12]

However, contact with Euro-Americans "brought unknown diseases—a strong element of unpredictability—and even though immunity to these diseases would likely be developing within one or two generations, the cultural traditions have no basis for identifying these causes of death and so they remain culturally unpredictable, which may help account for the anomie and other symptoms of distress—beyond those that would naturally be associated with being penned into a reservation." By using the Coale-Demeny model life tables, some suggestions can be made regarding pre-European-American-contact death rates. Weeks argues that "if we assume that the average Yakama was producing 5 live births (a little less than average for pre-modern women throughout the world), and that the population was growing slowly (0.5 percent per year—positive, but not widely perceptible in the short-term), then the life expectancy would had to have been about 30 years for women and about 28 for males." Under these conditions, females would have had a crude death rate around 38 per 1,000 in the Yakama population and males about 33 per 1,000. "The general fertility rate (babies per 1,000 women of reproductive ages) would be about 84." Furthermore, Weeks points out that if the above assumptions are correct then "the implied infant mortality rate is about 300 per 1,000 live births, and about 40 per cent of all deaths will be children under the age of 5." Weeks concludes by stating that if fertility were higher or growth slower, then death rates would have been higher. But if the growth rate were slower prior to contact, there would be a lower death rate.[13]

Contact with Euro–Americans brought on the Age of Pestilence that devastated native populations in the Northwest. The spread of disease and continuance of unhealthy conditions were made worse by government Indian policies designed to confine large numbers of diverse tribes and bands to single areas of land where the Office of Indian Affairs could control and convert them to white "civilization." A common hypothesis presented by historians argues that government Indian policies forced Native Americans from their traditional lands and ruined their economies. This occurred during the Age of Pestilence and Famine when the government of the United States concentrated a number of Indians on limited acres of tribal lands, designating these areas as reservations. The government expected Indian people to eke out a living as farmers (and later ranchers) on a small portion of their former landed estates, and in competition with other tribes and bands placed on the same reservation. These factors harmed native communities in many ways, particularly with regard to the health of people.[14]

During the late nineteenth and early twentieth centuries, Native Americans had to compete for their livelihood with non–Indians who resettled former Indian lands. These newcomers often changed the environment by ranching, farming, mining, irrigating, fencing, and road–building. Newcomers destroyed plant and animal habitats as well as natural resources such as game, fish, roots, berries, and timber. The results were disastrous for Indians in terms of diet and religion since they had a spiritual relationship to plants, animals, and places. Many times, government agents prevented Indians from hunting, fishing, and gathering off the reservation, in spite of treaty rights, because originally they wanted all Indians to become farmers tied to the soil. In the mid–twentieth century, officials of the Office of Indian Affairs often joined forces with state officials to prevent Yakama and other Indians from exercising their treaty rights to hunt, fish, and gather at all usual and accustomed areas on and off the reservation.[15]

Under the terms of the Yakama Treaty of 1855, the Indians secured for themselves their age–old right to fish, hunt, and gather. Although the treaty does not state specifically that the Yakama could fish off the reservation, it did state that they could fish at all usual and accustomed areas which included sites outside the reservation boundary.[16] All this was understood by

Indians and whites at the time of the Walla Walla Council. Prior to the establishment of the reservation, Yakama men, women, and children lived by following a seasonal round, fishing and gathering roots in the spring and summer, hunting in the fall and winter, and gathering berries in the summer and fall. Yakama and other Plateau Indians had practiced very limited farming prior to the establishment of reservations, since the earth held a bounty of natural foods that did not require cultivation. Agriculture on the Columbia Plateau had never been a major component of native economies.

The demand by the Office of Indian Affairs that the Yakama should become farmers was difficult at best and actually contrary to their spiritual beliefs which required them to eat specific foods at certain times of the year in order to celebrate and give thanks for these foods in holy feasts. In sum, the general policy of the Office of Indian Affairs was to force Yakama Indian people to remain on the reservation and make their livelihood through agriculture rather than by traditional means. Other agencies of the federal government aided in this effort by placing dams on Northwestern rivers and restricting the movement of Native Americans to hunting, fishing, and root grounds. Without the opportunity to hunt, fish, and gather as they had in previous years, the health of the Yakama Indians suffered, and people died as a result.[17]

Another factor that affected the health of Indians on the Yakama Reservation was housing. On most reservations, Indians had to live in non-traditional housing because of limited resources. Indians, like the Yakama, who were accustomed to traveling about in seasonal rounds were forced to remain in the same geographical area for large periods of time. This was a dangerous development and impaired the general health of Yakama people. Traditionally, Yakama lived in mat lodges, mat-covered tipis, and buffalo hide tipis. When they resided in their permanent village sites, they used their large A-framed mat lodges. When they began their seasonal round in the spring, they dismantled these lodges and moved to early root grounds using their tipis for housing. This system of seasonal rounds fostered hygiene, since the Yakama set up and dismantled their homes many times throughout the year and moved from place to place. Each time they moved, they cleaned their dwellings and policed their village sites.[18]

As a result of the reservation system, the Office of Indian Affairs encouraged Indians to remain on the reservation for most of the year. Resettlement of the Columbia Plateau by whites, the building of dams, and the destruction of the natural foods familiar to the Yakama brought about a change in life style and housing. Whites farmed, ranched, and logged many regions of the Columbia Plateau, modifying the environment, which was detrimental to Indians. Rather than moving about for a good portion of the year, the Yakama became confined to the reservation where they lived in mat lodges and small wood–framed dwellings throughout the year. These dwellings were overcrowded and unsanitary, most of them having dirt floors. The health of Yakama people suffered from inadequate sanitation, absence of clean ground water, polluted rivers from insecticides, and complete lack of any means for treating sewage. The change of housing among the Yakama contributed to their ill health, and as a consequence, the people became ill and died.[19]

When Indians became ill, the agency on the Yakama Reservation was poorly prepared to take care of them. Agents lacked adequate medicines, medical staff, sanitariums, and hospitals to care for the people. The Yakama Reservation encompassed over one million acres, and the lack of transportation for Indians and medical staff prevented people from receiving medical care. Traditional knowledge of curing procedures and medicinal plants was kept by elderly men and women, not herbal specialists. The elders were educated in the ways of the Yakama and commonly treated people before and after the establishment of the reservation. Traditional treatments for a number of medicinal problems continued to be used to fight eye problems, infections, and pain. However, Yakama people faced new biological enemies that did not respond to old treatments. Elders employed their knowledge but found it fairly ineffective in controlling tuberculosis, pneumonia, heart disease, measles, influenza, and syphilis.

Medicine men and women, trained to deal with different forms of "spirit sickness," were also unable to control these new diseases. It was a hopeless situation for people on the reservation, and Yakama society fell into a general anomie as the people were unable to heal themselves, control disease, or cope with reality resulting from the numerous illnesses and deaths suffered by friends and relatives on the reservation. The role of medicine men and women diminished over the years, in part because of the general breakdown in traditional culture resulting from the reservation system and American Indian policies. Before the arrival of whites, medicine men and women—especially midwives knowledgeable about pregnancies, nutrition, birth, delivery, and postpartum—healed people and provided preventive and curative information. These people had less influence after the arrival of "white man's diseases" that did not always subside when treated with traditional medicine.

Before the invasion of the Pacific Northwest by whites, Yakama people became ill from and died of spirit sickness, contact with powerful totems, violations of sacred places or procedures, and witchcraft. They also died of a number of physical causes, including infections, accidents, war, heart failure, cancer, etc. However, the white invasion brought with it the Age of Pestilence; its new diseases, environmental change, cultural dislocation, and social–political upheaval, all contributed to ill results. According to Abdel R. Omran, epidemiological transitions contributed to "the destruction of group cohesion, the rise of mental illness, crime, delinquency, drug dependency [including alcohol]," and cultural anomie. Moreover, he argues that populations were weakened by stress, hypertension, and suicidal tendencies.[20] As one person stated, "We get sickness from white man: measles, chickenpox, smallpox, whooping cough, flu, and all from white man."[21] Thus, the arrival of whites significantly changed the causes and cures of diseases that were previously known to the Indians. In addition, the reservation system and inadequacies of the Office of Indian Affairs generally contributed to the poor health of Native Americans on the Yakama Reservation. An analysis of the statistical data taken from the Death Certificates recorded for the various Indians on the Yakama Reservation supports these general assertions.

Unfortunately, no body of data regarding deaths on the Yakama Reservation is available for the years from 1859, when the United States created the Yakama Reservation, to 1888, when the agents collected the first death records for the Yakama Reservation. The censuses list the names of individuals by family, age, and sex. If a person died during the course of the year, the recording agent sometimes wrote "dead" or "died." It is unclear, however, in what year the person died, since censuses ran from 1 July to 30 June; nor do they state the primary or secondary causes of death. This is the extent of information regarding deaths that are sparsely provided in the early censuses. Because of the absence of detail data, no comparisons can be made mortality in the early nineteenth century when the Yakama were stricken by epidemics of smallpox, measles, and influenza and what would happen later. Death statistics for the period from 1888 and 1911 are poor, and the data kept by the Office of Indian Affairs between 1912 and 1923, although better, is not complete. However, the data available for the period after, the year when Indians became citizens of the United States and when Yakama agents responded to national Indian reforms, dramatically improved (figure 1.1). The present study is an examination of the available death data on the Yakama Reservation, particularly Death Certificates preserved by the Office of Indian Affairs after 1924. The study includes an analysis of causes and numbers of deaths on the reservation, particularly those of infants and small children. Admittedly, this is a narrow scholarly examination of one reservation, primarily using a single data source of 3,889 cases. Nevertheless, the data base assembled for this study is unique. It is the first ever assembled from Death Certificates on the Yakama Reservation, and it deals with a lengthy period of time. Although the data from 1888 to 1924 is weak, it represents a portion of the 3,899 cases kept at the National Archives for Yakama people and for this reason it is used in this study.

The work explores an aspect of Yakama history that has never been examined. The intent was to focus on reservation people, not urban Indians or those who filed Indian homesteads off the reservation, although many of the families who once owned homesteads or lived in urban areas joined their friends and relatives on the Yakama Reservation during the course of the nineteenth and twentieth centuries. This mortality study provides an in-depth work on one reservation over a period of seventy-six years, focusing on the social history of numerous Indian people living on a single reservation.[22] Although the agency letterbooks and reports to the Commissioner of Indian Affairs sometimes mentioned the number of deaths in any one year, agents of the Yakama Agency made no concerted effort to collect and preserve death registers until 1888. The present study is based on the 3,899 Death Certificates preserved in the National Archives, Pacific Northwest Region in Seattle, and the documents range over a period of time from 1888 to 1964.

The earliest death data collected by federal, county, and state officials from 1888 to 1923 is poor and suggests the lack of attention paid to the agency's mandated duty to collect and keep vital statistics. However, that data collected after 1924 is excellent, offering insights into the number and causes of death as well as other variables, including gender of the deceased, place of death, tribal affiliation, and blood quantum. The Yakama Agency kept Death Registers and Certificates which, incorrectly, would suggest that the Yakama experienced 1 death per year for the period from 1888 to 1905 and from 1907 to 1909. Yakama Agency officials preserved records indicating only 3 deaths in 1906 and 6 deaths in 1910. By any measure, these are low numbers, and they do not reflect the actual and, unfortunately, unknown number of deaths during the late nineteenth century and the early twentieth century. Some *Annual Reports of the Commissioners of Indian Affairs* provide the number of cases and deaths of a particular disease on the Yakama Reservation, but these are not used in this study due to the random and incomplete nature of these statistics, although they are helpful in an assessment of death in the late nineteenth and early twentieth centuries. They are not used to any degree because they are from a different data set, and this study is based on registers and certificates.[23]

Agents on the Yakama Reservation began collecting more information regarding deaths after 1910. This may have been the result of the Progressive Era in the United States and a renewed interest in the welfare of Native Americans, particularly by Commissioner of Indian Affairs Robert G. Valentine.[24] The trend to gather better data and record it might also have been linked to the General Allotment Act as it was applied to the Yakama Reservation in the early twentieth century. Under the terms of allotment, the United States divided a portion of the Yakama Reservation into individual allotments of 160-acre, 80-acre, and 40-acre parcels, depending on the age and marital status of individuals. In order to allot the reservation, agents required an accounting of all Indians living on or near the reservation, and agents conducted censuses on the Yakama

Reservation. Censuses also served as the basis for funding a particular reservation, so the more people agents listed on the censuses as Yakama living on the reservation, the more funding the agency received.

Death Certificates provided the Office of Indian Affairs with another means of tracking those Indians who were no longer within the Yakama population and who would not be allotted land. As a result of the Progressive Era and the General Allotment Act, the Office of Indian Affairs became involved in collecting better data on the Yakama Reservation, and the result was improved record keeping with regard to the Death Certificates. However, the best vital statistics on the Yakama Reservation came later, in the 1920s and 1930s, in response to another more profound reform movement. Even so, the data appears to be incomplete, particularly with regard to deaths for children under one year of age during the years between 1910 and early 1920s. Although inadequate, Death Certificates after 1910 indicate a new interest on the part of the Office of Indian Affairs to collect copies of Death Certificates; this led to the recording of a larger number of deaths (figures 1.1, 1.10). The Death Certificates after 1920 provide the most complete information of the deceased person's name, age, sex, and cause of death.[25]

Overall, the Office of Indian Affairs acquired the largest number of Death Certificates on the Yakama Reservation between 1924 and 1941, an era that corresponds with a major national reform movement in American Indian affairs.[26] As early as 1923, a committee of the United States Senate and members of the National Tuberculosis Association offered a study of tuberculosis among Native Americans. Under the chairmanship of George M. Kober, the committee investigated tuberculosis among many tribes, including the Yakama. Like many such studies, the report pointed out the problems associated with native people and tuberculosis, and recommended solutions to the epidemic that were not acted upon to any extent until the 1930s. Funding was the primary obstacle to facing tuberculosis on the reservations, in spite of widespread recognition that tuberculosis was a major health problem that affected Indians and non-Indians alike. Dr. Paul A. Turner of Washington stated that "The reporting of tuberculosis among Indians is not sufficient to answer the questions relating to increase or decrease."[27] Turner was correct since the *Annual Reports of the Commissioners of Indian Affairs* were often unclear about the number of cases of tuberculosis among the tribes in any one year from 1888 to 1920.

For example, in 1888, the report states that 1 Yakama died of scrofula but that there were 36 cases of the disease, and, in 1889, the report provides no details regarding deaths resulting from tuberculosis, stating only that "Scrofula and consumption are prevailing ailments."[28] The report of 1890 provides more data stating that there were 44 cases of tuberculosis on the Yakama Reservation and 41 cases of scrofula, but there is no information regarding the number of deaths caused by tuberculosis.[29] Between 1900 and 1904, the reports do not mention tuberculosis on the Yakama Reservation, and the disease is not featured as a major concern until after 1905. The reports are not complete regarding deaths resulting from tuberculosis on the reservation, although after 1905 they generally focus a good deal of attention to the disease. The Committee of the National Tuberculosis Association pointed out that the lack of sanitation was a primary problem on the reservation and that Indians needed to be educated about infectious diseases and ways to prevent disease. Another recommendation called for more hospitals and medical staff to identify the disease. A great deal of attention, the committee argued, should be placed on early detection of tuberculosis and repeated visits to doctors to check for the initial stages of infections. Furthermore, the committee recommended better housing for Indians, because Indian homes were overcrowded and unventilated. The committee cited housing as a "chief predisposing factor" in the spread of tuberculosis.[30] Homes, they maintained, also needed to be disinfected. Finally, committee members recommended better diets for Indians, citing food and diet as a factor affecting tuberculosis.[31]

The committee report included specific statistical data regarding deaths resulting from tuberculosis on the Yakama Reservation from 1911 to 1920. During this era, the Yakama reportedly suffered the largest number of deaths caused by tuberculosis in 1918 when 24 people died of the disease. The fewest number of deaths occurred in 1915 when 4 people died of tuberculosis on the Yakama Reservation. In contrast to this information, the Yakama Death Certificates indicate that only

13 (not 24) people died of tuberculosis in 1918 and that 17 people died of influenza that year, making influenza the leading cause of death in 1918. This is suggestive of the problem noted before of under reporting deaths through Death Certificates prior to 1924. According to the Report of the Committee of the National Tuberculosis Association, the average number of deaths caused by tuberculosis among the Yakama between 1911 and 1920 was 17 which indicates a larger number of deaths by the disease than provided in the Death Certificates. It also suggests that the tuberculosis epidemic began before 1924 when the Death Certificates indicate a huge jump in the number of deaths due to the disease. Statistics found in the report regarding tuberculosis deaths on the Yakama Reservation demonstrate convincingly that at least by 1911, when tuberculosis killed 21 people, the disease was already well established as a killer on the reservation. Tuberculosis had been a scourge of Yakama people much earlier, perhaps as early as the 1890s.[32] Although the National Tuberculosis Association joined forces with the United States Senate to investigate tuberculosis among native peoples and had made many insightful and useful recommendations, the government did not act on these suggestions for years. Instead, the government looked to another committee to research a wide variety of problems associated with American Indians, including the health of native peoples.

The next phase of the reform resulted in far-reaching changes in American Indian policy, and it is briefly presented below.[33] The reforms began, in part, as a result of a grant from John D. Rockefeller, Jr., to the Institute of Government Research—renamed the Brookings Institute. In 1926, the Institute launched a major investigation into the condition of Native Americans in terms of their health, education, and economy. In the same year, Lewis Meriam began his research which culminated in 1928 with the publication of *The Problem of Indian Administration*, commonly called *The Meriam Report*. The book was a revealing work which fueled the fires of national reformers. It examined many aspects of Indian life, providing a good deal of valuable information on Indian health and mortality.[34]

According to *The Meriam Report*, "taken as a whole practically every activity undertaken by the national government for the promotion of the health of the Indians is below a reasonable standard of efficiency."[35] Meriam also commented on the failure of the Office of Indian Affairs to meet minimum standards of governmental health care. "The health work of the Indian Service," Meriam wrote, "falls markedly below the standards maintained by the Public Health Service, the Veterans' Bureau, and the Army and the Navy, and those prescribed to the states by the national government in the administration of the . . . Maternity and Infancy Act." Furthermore, Meriam noted that a major problem in analyzing the health of Indians in the United States was the poor records collected and kept by the Indian Office. He reported that "for many years" the agencies "had rules and regulations requiring the collection and tabulation of vital statistics." After an exhaustive search through the records of several Indian agencies—including the Yakama Agency—Meriam found that "accurate figures based on reasonably complete records are not yet secured."[36]

In his landmark report, Meriam wrote that "many of the Indian deaths which occur on reservations" went unrecorded since "no report is made to the Indian Office." He maintained that when agents had collected Death Certificates, the information on the documents was "defective in that some of the essential items are missing." Meriam had studied Death certificates "with a view to learning the relative importance of various conditions in producing deaths," but he soon found that, on large numbers of the Death Certificates "a statement of the cause of death was missing."[37] This observation was made in reference to eleven reservations surveyed for their death records, none of which was the Yakama Reservation. Still, the statement is an accurate description of what happened there, as well. Meriam also contended that, since it was "a generally accepted axiom today that the quality of a service is accurately reflected in the completeness and accuracy of its records," it was factual to say that "the Indian Service has been weak."[38]

Meriam maintained correctly that "the statistics and records of medical activities at present are incomplete and unreliable."[39] Unfortunately, this is all too apparent in the records kept by the Yakama Indian Agency. The death records for the Yakama Reservation are incomplete, but they represent the only major data available on the subject and are valuable sources of information on the causes and numbers of deaths on one Indian reservation. The study began in the early 1920s when white reformers of Native American affairs in the United States demanded that the government investigate conditions on the reservations. The research committee led by Lewis Meriam was a direct result of their demands. The government published *The Meriam Report* in 1928, the year before the stock market crash and the onset of the Great Depression. Reform of American Indian affairs stalled until the election of Franklin D. Roosevelt who selected John Collier as his Commissioner of Indian Affairs. Collier kept this post until 1946, pressing forward with numerous national reforms in Indian affairs, including health, education, tribal government, and economic development.[40] This was part of the Indian New Deal. The statistics kept at the Yakama Agency show a dramatic improvement in numbers of deaths recorded and the completeness of the documents from 1924 to 1964, and this is a result of the national reforms, not an increased number of deaths on the reservation.

Because agents, doctors, and other employees working at the Yakama Agency did a poor job collecting documents and reporting deaths to county and state health officials, an accurate record of Death Certificates could not be made. Even as late as 1952, the Office of Indian Affairs reported that "no measure of the adequacy of death registration is available" because "cause-of-death reporting is slipshod and inaccurate." Dr. H. De Lien and J. Nixon Hadley pointed out that "Twenty years ago, it was a common practice to allow the reservation superintendent, who was not medically trained, to inscribe on the death certificate his surmise as to the cause of death."[41] In 1952, these authors argued that the agency

> doctor is frequently requested to assign a cause for a case that occurred 200 miles away and for which he has only hearsay evidence, sometimes supplemented by a previous hospital record. In many instances, he will indicate "cause unknown" but in others will hazard a "probably" such and such; and who can determine whether such a guess is or is not correct?[42]

Although Death Certificates collected with the help of agency physicians were flawed in relationship to cause of death, the data provided by these documents "represents the best available information of the person best-trained to make the determination, but is subject to an unknown percentage of error."[43]

Federal and state officials were derelict in their duties to collect accurate and complete Death Certificates for several reasons. For one, white officials working for the state and federal governments were dealing with Indians, people who some non-Indians considered backward, uncivilized, barbaric, and savage. To some, Indians were the "Vanishing Race," and some whites viewed Indian deaths as a natural consequence of interfacing with "advanced civilization." Some agents, including well-meaning Christians, viewed the death of Native Americans under their care as an embarrassment to themselves, the Indian Office, and the nation. If the non-native public of the United States knew the actual number of Indian deaths, they might have demanded greater and more far-reaching reforms than they did in the early twentieth century.

On the Yakama Reservation, none of the agents serving from 1888 to 1910 considered the collection of vital statistics regarding Indian deaths to be a priority, or if they did, they did not convey their conviction to those responsible for collecting data. Agents and their employees managed all of the business associated with the reservation, and they did not focus their attention on recording vital statistics. Perhaps they were preoccupied with issues involving agriculture, irrigation, fishing, education, road building, timber harvests, land allotments, law enforcement, trade, and other such matters. They were busy "civilizing" and Christianizing Indians as well. Agents were a part of a huge bureaucracy that dealt in paper—writing letters, taking censuses, completing forms, and filing reports. They likely did not champion the task of tracking Indian deaths, especially on a land base as rural and as large as the Yakama Reservation with a population roughly ranging from 2,000 to 3,000 people (figure 1.7).[44] Furthermore, some employees of the Indian Affairs Office felt that the duty of dealing with vital statistics was one that involved counties and states, not agencies. Transportation and communication systems were not well developed on the reservation, making it difficult for county, state, and federal officials to learn about deaths that occurred some distance from agency headquarters at Fort Simcoe or Toppenish. Between 1888 and 1910, officials of the Indian Office made little effort to record deaths in any area of the reservation, including that region surrounding Fort Simcoe.[45]

In addition to governmental inefficiency, Indians themselves contributed to the lack of information regarding deaths within their own communities. Sometimes long distances separated Yakama people from the agency. Poor transportation and communication systems worked against any effort on their part to report deaths. However, it is important to note that many—if not most—Yakama people resented the government of the United States for its control of nearly every aspect of tribal affairs. Few Yakama were interested in cooperating with whites by sharing their most personal grief with agents who had dictated policy to them since 1855. This was particularly true regarding parents who lost fetuses and infants, since families and friends quietly mourned these deaths in their own fashion, burying the children without notifying agents. When deaths occurred, one of the last things on the minds of Yakama families was to notify county, state, or agency officials so that white bureaucrats could record an Indian death. To have done so would have been to participate in the white man's bureaucracy which some Yakama held in contempt.

As a result of many factors, Death Certificates do not represent the full range of deaths that occurred on the Yakama Reservation from 1888 to 1964. Federal and state officials sometimes learned of the death of elders, since their funerals brought large numbers of Indians to a particular area to mourn, Usually, the death of an important man or woman resulted in an outpouring of gifts and participation by larger Northwestern Indian communities. The death of fetuses, infants, or children, did not attract as many people, particularly those from other reservations, and some of these deaths and burials went unnoticed and unrecorded by the state. Still, a large portion of the known deaths were those of children, which leaves one only to surmise the number of fetal, infant, and childhood deaths never recorded by the government (figures 1.6, 3.5, 3.6, 3.7, 3.8).

As has been said, despite their being incomplete, Death Certificates and Registers for the Yakama Indian Reservation offer the best information available regarding deaths among Yakama people from 1888 to 1964. Some individual family members kept oral and written accounts of deaths in their families, but copies of the Washington state Death Certificates kept for the Yakama Agency are the most complete recorded information available regarding deaths on the reservation during this seventy-six-year period. This study is based on these documents, with individual descendants as the unit of analysis. It is an attempt at a census, rather than a sample, of Yakama deaths, since it considers the death of every person whose death was recorded through Death Certificates or Registers. The study takes into account eight variables found on the death certificates: year of death, age at death, gender, cause of death, place of death, tribal affiliation, ward, and blood quantum. The first four variables are most important to the work, and they therefore receive far more attention than the final four.

Univariate Analysis of Yakama Death Certificates

The data used in the statistical analysis of Yakama deaths from 1888 to 1964 is based primarily on the Death Certificates. Each of the variables found in these documents is discussed below. Some of these variables proved to be important in an understanding of death over time on the Yakama Reservation, while others were not. In addition to the data taken from the Death Certificates, the study offers some comparisons regarding death among non-Indian populations. Comparative data regarding crude death rates, fetal death rates, and infant mortality rates are presented, comparing the Yakama population with the white population of the United States, non-white population of the United States, African Americans in the United States, and the general population of Washington. These are to provide a comparative framework from which to examine Yakama statistical data. Readers should recognize the limitations of comparing a small Yakama population with larger populations and note that moving averages are provided to enhance such comparisons by smoothing out the data. Fluctuations in the data are often more erratic in smaller populations than in larger ones, and this is often the case with the Yakama data. Therefore, some moving averages are provided to view the data over periods of time. It is hoped that the comparative study will help scholars assess the relative importance of specific causes of death among the Yakama as compared to other populations within the United States.[46]

Year of Death

One of the variables found on the Death Certificates was the year of death, and it was measured as an interval-level variable. Death Certificates nearly always contained the year of death, and so most of this data was complete since it was recorded regularly in the documents. As noted earlier, The data for the early years is incomplete. Only 1 death per year is reported for the years from 1888 to 1905 and for the years 1907 and 1909. This is the lowest number of deaths per year recorded in the data set. The data between 1888 and 1910 is weak and does not represent accurately the number of deaths on the Yakama Reservation, but it is included with the other years because together the data offers insights into deaths for a lengthy period of time.

The highest number of recorded deaths occurred in 1928 when the agency recorded 229 deaths. This was the year that the government of the United States released *The Meriam Report*, and the large number of deaths recorded on the Yakama Reservation during this year was probably linked with the nationwide demand for better record keeping by the Indian Office and the publication of the report. Indeed, during the period from 1924 to 1941, government officials reported more deaths and agents preserved more Death Certificates than at any other time during the seventy-six year period under discussion. During the seventeen year period between 1924 and 1941, they recorded a total of 2,323 deaths (60 percent). The large number of deaths may have been a result of a response to the Great Depression, but it is more likely that it represented a reaction to national reforms in the Office of Indian Affairs and the leadership of John Collier as Commissioner of Indian Affairs.

The number of Yakama deaths declined dramatically during the 1940s because of the eradication of tuberculosis and gastrointestinal disorders. The incidence of tuberculosis may have waned as a cause of death as a result of a natural decline of the disease, a pattern it has followed throughout human history. Simply put, tuberculosis had run its course although it had not

completely disappeared.[47] It also declined, along with gastrointestinal disorders, because of advances in public health and
general, medical practices, sanitation programs, and improved
income. The number of deaths also decreased due to political
changes, changes that turned the nation's attention to World
War II and the production of materiel to support the war
effort. Many Yakama went off to fight while others, including
women, remained behind to work in war industries. The war
was a watershed in Yakama history epidemiologically and
nutritionally. During the war, most Yakama became wage
earners, using their cash earnings to purchase refined foods.
Fewer Yakama could hunt, fish, and gather as they had in the
past, so many Yakama turned to processed foods. In addition,
housing, medical care, medicines, sanitation, and public health
improved in the 1940s. World War II brought many Yakama
into the geo-political sphere of the United States, lessening
feelings of alienation. All of these factors influenced a major
change in the primary causes of death on the reservation from
contagious diseases to man-made problems such as heart
disease, cancer, accidents, diabetes, and accidental deaths.

After World War II, the overall number of deaths on the
Yakama Reservation decreased significantly for several reasons.
Mortality declined because of better public health, sanitation,
housing, food, medicines (including antibiotics), and increases
in family incomes.[48] Preston and Haines have remarked that
child mortality was high in the late nineteenth century, not
because of neglect or an absence of resources, but because
people lacked the knowledge of how to prevent infectious
disease. Nevertheless, it is significant that by the 1940s, the
Yakama had gained both resources and the knowledge with
which to combat such diseases. And by the 1950s, the Public
Health Service had taken over health care on the reservation
and ended the relative neglect of health care given to Yakama
people during the first half of the twentieth century.[49] However, Hunn was "puzzled by the sharp drop in reported deaths
after 1940." He noted that "While improved medical treatment
and hygiene might account for some reduction, this is also a
time when the total base population is growing rapidly, and in
general, the larger the population, the more deaths."[50] Hunn is
correct in pointing out the drop in the number of deaths
reported after 1940, which may have something do with

national events. Furthermore, during the early part of that decade, the United States turned its attention overseas where the Second World War raged on many fronts. Washington officials working within the Office of Indian Affairs may have placed less emphasis on the collection of vital statistics on the reservations, particularly statistics that would have required greater governmental resources to combat death and disease. The decline in the number of Death Certificates during the 1940s may have been linked to political changes in the federal government during the war and immediately afterward when the nation was more preoccupied with the spread of communism than the collection of vital statistics on Indian reservations. There may have been a change in reporting practices of the Yakama Agency after 1940, which, in part, also accounts for smaller number of reported deaths between 1940 and 1964.[51]

Age at Death

The second variable coded in the study was the person's age at death, and county and state officials usually recorded the person's age on the Death Certificates. Between 1888 and 1964, the mean age of death on the Yakama Reservation was 33 with a standard deviation of 5. For females the mean age of death was 35 with a standard deviation of 9, and for males the mean age was 31 with a standard deviation of 6.5. Age at death was coded as an interval-level variable from 0 to 99, with 0 representing the death of those children under one year of age and stillborn infants, and 99 representing persons dying at 99 years of age or older. Only a few individuals were reported as dying at 100 years of age or older, and most of these were males.

It is important to note that the modal age of death was under one year of age, a circumstance common in many world populations. A total of 737 or 19 percent of all deaths in the population from the 1910s to the 1960s were among Yakama fetuses and infants that died before they were one year of age (figures 1.6, 3.10). This is the largest number of deaths for any age group. A total of 106 fetal deaths(14 percent) were reported, 631 of the deaths (86 percent) were among the infant population. A total of 235 (6 percent) children died between the age of one and two years of age, while 112 (3 percent) died between the ages of two and three. The number of reported deaths decreased as children got older. A total of 67 (2 percent) children died during their third year, 62 (2 percent) during their fourth year, and 35 (1 percent) during their fifth year. Roughly one third of all deaths on the Yakama Reservation between 1888 and 1964 were those of children less than six years of age (figures 3.6, 3.7, 3.8). The high number of infant and childhood deaths on the Yakama Reservation is similar to that found in some countries of Africa, Asia, and Latin America.

The distribution is skewed to the right due to the high number of deaths among infants and children under six years of age. As a result of the large number of deaths among fetuses, infants, and children, the study focuses on childhood deaths in the analysis, providing an examination of different age groups. In addition, the work examines those age categories of children of one year of age and those two to six years of age.

Gender

Gender was measured in the study as a nominal variable. Between 1888 and 1964, a total of 1,922 females died (49 percent), while 1,960 males died (50 percent) which is a fairly even and normal split in the population. A total of 17 Death Certificates did not include the person's gender. The analysis of the data demonstrates that while females and males generally died of the same major causes of death, there were significant differences between male and female death rates with regard to various causes (figure 3.11). For example, cancer, meningitis, stroke, natural causes, and childbirth were among the ten leading causes of death among Yakama females, but none of these causes appear in the ten major causes of death among males. In the same way, premature birth and alcohol-related deaths were two of the foremost causes of death among Yakama males, but these two causes of death were not among the ten leading causes of death among females. The impact of gender on cause of death will be discussed more fully in a later section.

Cause of Death

One of the most important variables in the study was cause of death, and it was a nominal variable. Numeric codes were developed for each distinct cause of death, and cases were coded accordingly. In cases where more than one cause of death was listed for an individual, the case was assigned the numeric code corresponding to the first or primary cause of death listed on the Death Certificate. Since the study begins in 1888, no attempt is made to analyze deaths prior to this date. Unfortunately, data for deaths during the Age of Pestilence of the eighteenth and nineteenth centuries are not available for the Yakama, so no comparisons can be made among the causes of death in those centuries. It is known from the historical literature that smallpox from trading vessels arrived in the Northwest in 1775, and it came up the Missouri River, spreading death in 1782-83, 1801, 1824-25. This disease killed a large but unknown number of Indians in the Northwest as did "fever and ague." The "Cold Sickness," or influenza also killed a number of Indians in epidemics, and in 1847 a measles epidemic ravaged the Cayuse and other Indians of the Inland Northwest.[52] No analysis is made of these causes of death among Yakama people prior to 1888, since they are not within the scope of the data set used in this study.

Omran has pointed out that "scattered accounts of epidemics leave no doubt of their existence in the 18th and parts of the 19th century." These epidemics included "intermittent fever (now malaria), typhoid, influenza, measles, parotitis, scarlatina, smallpox, syphilis, thrush, whooping cough, and yellow fever. Consumption (tuberculosis), pneumonia, and bronchitis were grouped under respiratory diseases."[53] Epidemics of some of these spread among Plateau Indians, but no accurate records exist regarding the numbers of people who died of these scourges. Moreover, during the era of this study, tuberculosis, influenza, pneumonia, bronchitis, and whooping cough were major killers of Yakama people. Yet information taken from Death Certificates indicated that these were only 5 of the 87 causes of death coded from the Yakama data base. By 1888 smallpox and measles were insignificant killers of Yakama people, but other causes of death—particularly tuberculosis and pneumonia—continued to plague the people, bringing death throughout the early twentieth century.

The present work does not deal with all causes of death among the Yakama but concentrates primarily on the ten leading causes of death in the general population and the top five causes of death among infants and children. Several causes of death occurred only a few times in the data set, including "arthritis," "bad cold," "diphtheria," "epilepsy," "fever," "gonorrhea," "rickets," and "carbuncle." The minor causes of death will not be addressed in the work. Unfortunately, of the 3,899 cases reported in the data set, the cause of death of 1,082 (28 percent) individuals is unknown, unrecorded, or illegible in the Death Certificates. Several of the Death Certificates simply did not include the cause of death or included the statement "Not Known."

Several other Death Certificates had a handwritten cause of death, but the writing was not legible. If the statement was illegible, the person's death was coded as unknown. However, every effort was made to read these with a magnifying glass and in consultation with colleagues. The large number of unknown, unrecorded, and illegible statements regarding the cause of death represents poor or careless record keeping on the part of county and state officials or agents and reservation doctors who were required by state law to keep vital statistics and aid in the collection and preservation of accurate statistics. The unknown, unrecorded, and illegible causes of death will not be addressed in the narrative, but mention of the number and percentage of these deaths is provided in end notes. The percentages given in the analysis are based on known deaths and variables, without consideration for the unknown deaths.

In coding causes of death, the study provides a single "cause" for the death of each individual. In some cases, county and state officials recorded the primary and secondary causes on Death Certificates. In such cases, the author coded only the primary causes but made note of secondary causes in the data set. For example, if the person died of pneumonia but also had tuberculosis, which probably contributed to the onset of pneumonia, the cause of death was coded as pneumonia, not tuberculosis. Likewise, if a person died in an automobile accident but was intoxicated, the death was coded as an automobile accident but it was noted in the margins of the code sheet that the accident was alcohol-related.[54] Thus, secondary causes of death were recorded in the data set but they are not the main focus of this work.

The rankings of the causes of death are provided below. This is followed by a brief description of each cause. Within the entire population on the Yakama Reservation, tuberculosis (N = 619/28 percent of all deaths) was the most common cause of death during the seventy-six-year period, followed by pneumonia (N = 566/26 percent). The third leading cause of death was heart diseases (N = 325/15 percent), followed by miscellaneous accidents (N = 145/7 percent). The fifth leading cause of death on the Yakama Reservation was gastrointestinal disorders (N = 124/6 percent), and the sixth cause of death was automobile accidents (N = 122/5.5 percent). Influenza (N = 104/5 percent) was the seventh leading cause of death, and cancer (N = 82/3 percent) was the eighth. Premature births (N = 64/3 percent) and senility and old age (N = 57/3 percent) rounded out the ninth and tenth most common causes of death among females and males on the Yakama Reservation.[55]

The analysis examines crude death rates per 100,000 in the population among different American populations for selected years (figure 3.12). Comparisons of crude death rates among the Yakama and other populations due to different causes of death are provided. Comparisons of the Yakama to other populations prior to the mid-1910s cannot be made, because the Yakama death records are so sparse. However, comparisons are made regarding causes of death, crude death rates, fetal death rates, and infant mortality rates among diverse populations in the United States for those years between 1920 and 1960. Comparisons are made between the Yakama population, the African American population of the United States, populations in Washington state, and white/non-white populations of the United States. In addition, the death rates for infants and small children are provided with comparisons to the general population of the United States.

Fetal and infant mortality rates per 1,000 are also offered in comparison with those of other American populations (figures 1.6, 3.5). These rates are calculated for all years in which data is available.[56] Data was available to calculate infant mortality rates for most years between 1914 and 1964. The infant mortality rate for the Yakama is compared in the analysis with whites and "non-whites" or the combined populations of Latinos, Asian Americans, Native American, African Americans, and other "non-whites" in the population of the United States. "Non-whites" is the designation given to all people of color, and it is used in this study to conform with the statistics provided by the United States government. The comparisons demonstrate that the infant mortality rate on the Yakama Reservation was nearly always many times greater than that of the white and non-white populations of the United States as well as the population of Washington state during most of the twentieth century until the 1960s. In addition to providing death rates of fetuses, infants, and children, and data on the ten leading causes of death the study focuses on the rate of death suffered by Yakama people and other populations in the United States. These causes of death are described below in order of their prominence among Yakama people for the period from 1888 to 1964. Included is a discussion of tuberculosis, pneumonia, and other significant killers of Yakama Indians.

Tuberculosis

The most frequently recorded cause of death from 1888 to 1964 was tuberculosis (N = 619/28 percent), and it preyed on the Yakama until its near eradication in the 1940s (figure 1.2, 1.4). Usually the disease develops slowly and, historically, it was difficult to diagnose. Indeed, as Barbara Gutmann Rosenkrantz has noted, "Not even a well-trained physician would diagnose tuberculosis without an X-ray and other procedures to distinguish between the coughs, sputum, and breath-sounds that different pulmonary diseases have in common."[57] Tuberculosis is caused by airborne bacilli which spread from one person to the next. It was prevalent on the Yakama Reservation because of abject poverty suffered within a concentrated native population. Confinement on the reservation and living in substandard and unsanitary housing with no public health contributed to the spread of tuberculosis. The lack of medical care, medicines, hospitals, sanitariums, and dwindling natural food resources off the reservation kept Indians in a state of ill health. Processed foods were not as nutritious as traditional foods. Confinement to the reservation led to permanent homes that were less sanitary than temporary mat lodges and tipis that were continually built and re-built throughout the year. The reservation system encouraged poverty, ill health, depression, and death. Indians had little knowledge of air-borne infectious diseases or how to prevent the spread of disease. Those Yakama between the ages of 15 and 29 suffered the most deaths resulting from tuberculosis on the reservation.

The reservation also offered a breeding ground for bacilli and viruses that caused tuberculosis, pneumonia, gastrointestinal disorders, and other maladies. Cows can also carry tubercle bacteria (*mycobacterium. Bovus*), and the disease may be transmitted through milk, although this was not likely a major cause of tuberculosis among the Yakama because the people did not drink large quantities of cow's milk, owing in part to allergies to it. Tuberculosis is characterized by a dry cough accompanied by phlegm, pus, and blood. Victims usually suffer fever, fatigue, and loss of appetite. Persons afflicted with the disease often lose weight and may develop lumps in their body. Tuberculosis can attack various parts of the body, including bones, brains, and kidneys. However, most often it spreads to the lungs where the bacilli multiply, inflaming the tissue of the affected area.

Tuberculosis acts in two stages, the first being a bacilli attack on a particular part of the body (most often the lungs initially), which is then counter-attacked by the body's defenses.[58] For several months, the body's antibodies surround and attack the bacteria, but generally some of the bacilli escape and move through the blood to other areas. Antibodies corral the bacteria in the new area, and this process may last for months. Antibodies simply contain bacteria, but they do not kill them. For this reason, the tubercle bacilli can become active at any point. This is particularly true if the person becomes undernourished, weak, or ill from another disease, which was a common condition on the reservation. Thus, in the death records for the Yakama, county and state officials sometimes recorded that, in addition to tuberculosis, people were assigned secondary causes of death. Secondary causes included heart disease, syphilis, influenza, and meningitis.

The second phase of the disease is often referred to in the Death Certificates as "consumption" (pulmonary tuberculosis).[59] The body's defenses are not sufficient to contain bacilli, and they begin to grow at an alarming rate. If the lungs become infected, the person has trouble breathing. If the tuberculosis spreads to other parts of the body, the disease can become active there as well, particularly if the person is weakened by the primary attack of the disease or has contracted another illness.[60] Tuberculosis was the principal killer of Yakama Indians between 1888 and 1964, and it was an important disease among Native Americans in the United States until the 1940s. Tuberculosis was listed as the cause of death for 619 (28 percent) of Yakama people. It probably killed many others whose cause of death was listed as "unknown," and it certainly killed untold numbers of Indian people on the Yakama Reservation between 1890 and 1924—before the Office of Indian Affairs began collecting Death Certificates in earnest.[61] The disease ravaged the Yakama population until the 1940s when a dramatic change occurred. During World War II, the Yakama experienced a radical drop in mortality due to a decrease in the number of deaths caused by tuberculosis. Significantly, this decline occurred before the Public Health Service took over Indian health and before advances were made by Selman Waksman in finding antibiotics that would fight the tubercle bacilli. Thus the decline in the number of Yakama deaths resulting from tuberculosis was due to several factors including better public health, housing, sanitation, isolation, and knowledge about the spread and prevention of the disease. In addition, the decline in the number of tuberculosis deaths resulted from increased income and a natural decline of the disease.[62] Deaths caused by tuberculosis decreased sufficiently so that during the period from 1950 to 1964, it killed only 13 Yakama people.

Sometimes deaths by tuberculosis were complicated by secondary infections of pneumonia or a malady identified by physicians as pneumonitis. However, in most cases, officials recording Yakama deaths through the Death Certificates often provided specific descriptions of the disease, including "pulmonary tuberculosis," "tuberculosis of bones," and "glandular tuberculosis." Sometimes people with tuberculosis suffered complications brought on by secondary infections, including "tuberculosis and pneumonia," "tuberculosis and meningitis," and "tuberculosis and syphilis." Tuberculosis seemed to have been nearly eradicated in the United States by the 1950s, "and the number of TB cases steadily decreased until 1986, when an increase was noted; TB has continued to rise since."[63] This rise in the number of tuberculosis cases is closely associated with HIV infections and the AIDS epidemic. Tuberculosis was a devastating disease, and it was the leading cause of death on the Yakama Reservation.[64]

Pneumonia

Like tuberculosis, pneumonia (figure 1.5 and 3.4) flourished on the reservation because of poor housing, inadequate diets, lack of public health and sanitation, and insufficient medicine and medical staff (N = 566/26 percent). Pneumonia is usually caused by viral or bacterial infections, but it can also result from chemicals like poison gas. However, unless a Yakama individual was exposed to gas in Word War I, it is unlikely that this was a factor causing pneumonia on the Yakama Reservation. Pneumonia may be brought on by an influenza virus, or it may be caused by bacteria. Pneumonia caused by viruses are far more difficult to treat because they do not respond to antibiotics. For Indians lacking natural immunities, sanitation, public health, and suffering from malnutrition, depression, or other diseases, pneumonia was extremely deadly.

In general, two major types of bacterial or viral pneumonia exist: lobar pneumonia and bronchopneumonia. Lobar pneumonia is characterized by an inflammation of one lobe of one lung that can spread to other lobes. In bronchopneumonia, the inflammation begins in the bronchioles and bronchi—airways—and spreads to tissues in one or both lungs. The most common form of bacterial pneumonia is streptococcus pneumonia, although other forms of bacterial pneumonia include hemophilus influenzae, legionella pneumonphilia, staphylococcus aureus, and others.[65] Pneumonia is commonly characterized by inflammation of the lungs, but it includes many other inflammations. Part or all of one lung might be affected or both lungs can contract pneumonia. Individuals with the disease often cough, exhibit high fevers, suffer chills, sweat profusely, and complain of chest pains. They may be short of breath while resting, and they may cough phlegm that contains blood. Sometimes children with pneumonia have a blue tint to their skin and lips. People with the disease sometimes suffer delirium, and in severe cases, they die. This is particularly true of patients with tuberculosis, heart disease, cancer, and bronchitis. This can also be the case of someone who has had a stroke. Thus, pneumonia may be diagnosed as the immediate cause of death when the person was stricken by some other illness first.[66]

Many Death Certificates indicate that the person simply died of pneumonia, but in some cases, the documents describe the deaths as "pneumonia and influenza," "pulmonary pneumonia," "pneumonia following measles," and "lobar pneumonia." Of the people on the Yakama Reservation who died between 1888 and 1964, a total of 566 (26 percent) succumbed to pneumonia. Pneumonia was the foremost cause of death among Yakama infants and children under six years of age. Many more Yakama male infants died of pneumonia than females, but this is common among infants in general. According to Charles B. Clayman, writing for the American Medical Association in the *Encyclopedia of Medicine*, pneumonia "is more common in males, during infancy and old age." However, Clayman does not explain why.[67] One eminent professor of ethnic studies, has suggested that more male infants than female infants died of pneumonia because of child abuse, but there is no social, cultural, or scientific evidence to support such an assertion.[68] During the 1940s and 1950s, pneumonia continued to cause death on the Yakama Reservation, at the very time that tuberculosis declined as the major cause of death. During the fourteen year period from 1950 through 1964, pneumonia caused the death of 125 Yakama people. A total of 22 percent of all deaths caused by pneumonia occurred during the last fourteen years covered by this study.[69] Although the Yakama population experienced many advances in public health, sanitation, diet, housing, and education, they continued to suffer from pneumonia throughout the twentieth century.

Heart Diseases

Heart diseases (figure 3.13) of all kinds, including heart disorders, diseases of the valves, heart attacks, heart failure, congenital heart disease, and others, represent the third leading cause of death among the Yakama during the late nineteenth and early twentieth centuries (N = 325/15 percent). Tobacco use was not a common practice among Yakama before World War II, and therefore smoking did not contribute greatly to heart disease prior to the 1950s. Instead, heart disease is linked to diet which changed dramatically during the course of the twentieth century from fish, game, native fruits, and vegetables to processed foods, including government commodities. According to Popkin, changes in diet are related to "modernization" and shift patterns of mortality. One such dramatic change among Yakama people was the rise in heart disease after World War II which, in part, was likely the result of changing diet and nutritional value of foods eaten by Yakama after the war.[70]

Nutritional and dietary changes also affected pregnant mothers and their children. "Many females," according to Omran, "developed pelvic deformities [as infants and children] with rickets which led to later difficulties in childbirth and higher rates of maternal death."[71] Poor diets weakened the health of many people, including pregnant mothers whose children were sometimes born with heart diseases. Heart attack was a major cause of death within this category and is characterized by blockage caused by blood clots in coronary arteries, which cuts off the supply of blood to one region of the heart muscle and damages that part of the heart. Generally the clot is caught in the blood vessel because the artery has an atheroma, or fatty deposit, that narrows and restricts the flow of blood. Persons suffering from a heart attack have severe angina in the chest, neck, jaw, arms, and stomach. They may also experience shortness of breath, chills, fainting, nausea, sweating, and dizziness. A heart attack may be fatal if it impedes the electrical impulses that regulate the heart or if damage to the heart is severe.[72]

Another common aspect of heart disease affecting Yakama Indians was heart failure. Weakened heart muscle or valves can impair the pumping of the heart, making the organ inefficient. When this happens, heart failure occurs. When the heart cannot pump a normal amount, blood collects in the vessels and flows either into the lungs or other parts of the body, overloading the areas with excess blood. Heart failure stresses the entire body, and it can be fatal. When a woman is pregnant, her heart must work harder than normal. If the mother has a heart disorder, including a murmur, complications during the prenatal period or childbirth might prove fatal.[73]

Babies also suffered from congenital heart disorders or abnormalities of the heart at the time of birth. Congenital heart disease can be caused if the mother has an infection or German measles (rubella). A fetus may develop heart problems during the first three months after conception, and the cause may not be known.[74] Congenital heart disease can be fatal to an infant, but between 1888 and 1964, government officials recording Yakama deaths reported that only 2 percent of all children who died between birth and age five died of heart disease. However, heart disease was the third largest killer of all Indians on the Yakama Reservation during the seventy-six year period. During the 1940s and 1950s, while tuberculosis declined rapidly as a major cause of death among Yakama people, heart disease became the leading killer on the reservation. Between 1950 and 1964, heart disease claimed the lives of 127 people. Of all Yakama who died of heart disease during the last fourteen years included in this study, 29 percent died as a result of heart disease. Washington state officials recorded the deaths of Yakama from heart disease in many ways, including "heart failure," "arteriosclerosis," "organic heart disease," "pulmonary edema," and "pulmonary hemorrhage." In addition, sometimes officials reported secondary causes of death associated with heart disease, including "heart disease and premature childbirth," "heart and renal disease," and "heart disease and pleurisy." Heart disease was a significant cause of death on the Yakama Reservation, particularly after 1950 when it became the leading cause of death.[75]

Miscellaneous Accidents

Miscellaneous accidents (figure 3.1 and 3.2) was the fourth most frequent killer of the Yakama, and many accidents were coded in this category (N = 145/7 percent), except those brought about from automobile accidents. It was an important category of death for the general population of Yakama people throughout the twentieth century and remains so today. Accidental deaths occurred from poisoning, falls, drowning, and electrocution. Often the Death Certificates are explicit about this cause of death, including statements such as "thrown by a horse," "burned to death," "fall from wagon," "blood poisoning from a nail," "run over by train," "logging accident," "fractured skull from dynamite," "drowning," "accidental gunshot wound," and "rattlesnake bite." Miscellaneous accidents were an important cause of death among children and adults.[76]

Gastrointestinal Disorders

The fifth major cause of death in the general Yakama population was gastrointestinal disorders (figure 3.14). Problems of the stomach, intestines, and other organs of the digestive tract proved fatal to adults and children alike, particularly if infections developed (N = 124/6 percent). Prior to the 1930s, antibiotics were not available to the Yakama, and they were sometimes in short supply during the years following their introduction on the reservation (figure 3.15). Although the digestive tract naturally contains necessary and vital bacteria, harmful bacteria sometimes invade the body where they can multiply rapidly, infecting the gut wall and enter the bloodstream. Dangerous bacteria can spread to other areas of the body, including other parts of the digestive system, and they can prove harmful or deadly to a person.

Nearly all infections of the digestive tract are caused by bacteria, and infants can ingest bacteria from unsterilized bottles, clothes, and unclean parts of another's body, particularly unclean breasts and unwashed hands. Infants are especially vulnerable to bacilli contracted from fecal material. People infected with gastrointestinal disorders usually exhibit one or more symptoms. They may experience general intestinal and abdominal pains, cramps, vomiting, fever, and diarrhea. Usually, people suffering from gastrointestinal disorders will become thirsty, but they are often unable to keep fluids in their stomachs because of vomiting. The malady is complicated by diarrhea which contributes significantly to the person's state of dehydration.[77] Disorders of the stomach, intestines, and other parts of the digestive tract accounted for 124 deaths in the general Yakama population. Officials recorded deaths resulting from gastrointestinal disorders in many different ways, including "stomach trouble," "bowel trouble," "intestinal obstruction," "enterocolitis," "gastroenteritis," "cholelia-thiasis," and "accute [sic] enteritis."[78]

Automobile Accidents

Automobile accidents (figure 3.3) were the sixth leading cause of death on the reservation (N = 122/5.5 percent). This is remarkable in one respect, since most Yakama did not own motor vehicles until the 1930s and 1940s. Automobile accidents are common today near Indian reservations and tribal lands, in part, because city, county, and federal officials historically have placed a low priority on preventive road work, signals, signs, and lighting near Indian lands. Officials in border towns near reservations and state officials are notorious for ignoring areas well traveled by Native American drivers, often circulating tasteless jokes about losing Indians to automobile accidents. This may have been a factor in the number of deaths suffered by Indians on or near the Yakama Reservation. Descriptions discussing death by automobile and truck accidents in the Death Certificates are not detailed. Most of them simply state "Injuries suffered in auto accident" or "auto accident." However, some of the Death Certificates state that the person died by "auto accident due to alcohol," "Injuries from auto accident/alcohol," or "Injuries, auto accident, drowning," "drowned, auto accident," "injuries from auto accident," "skull fracture—car accident," "burning auto," and "brain damage—auto accident." The first automobile fatality suffered by a Yakama person traveling inside a car occurred in 1924, but the vast majority of deaths by vehicular accidents occurred between 1940 and 1964.[79]

Influenza

The seventh leading cause of death on the Yakama Reservation was influenza (figure 1.2)—a disease often identified as flu (N = 104/5 percent). Many varieties of influenza viruses exist, and they are continually evolving with new strains developing all the time. Influenza is an airborne disease that generally spreads when an infected person coughs or sneezes. The virus enters the body through the upper respiratory system—the nose and mouth—and it frequently travels into the lungs. Within days after contact, a person may show symptoms such as sneezing, coughing, sore throat, chills, chest pains, head and muscular aches, and high fever.[80] Medical doctors and state recording officials sometimes linked influenza and pneumonia, but most often they recorded "influenza" as the primary and only cause of death, stipulating "Spanish influenza," "intestinal influenza," influenza since birth," and "grippe." At times influenza was linked to other causes of death, and some Death Certificates state that Yakama people died of "Spanish influenza and tuberculosis," "influenza and pneumonia," "flu and senility," and "influenza and choletithitis."[81]

Epidemics of influenza occurred on the Yakama Reservation, spreading to many Indians and killing some. Historically, influenza was a major killer of Native Americans in general and of Northwestern Indians in particular. It was sometimes labeled the "Cold Sickness" by white observers, and it devastated entire villages along the lower Columbia River. In 1827 and 1829, Northwestern Indians probably suffered from influenza. But worse yet was "fever and ague" which flourished in the 1830s and has been identified by Robert Boyd as malaria.[82] The disease or diseases caused a horrible epidemic which traveled from the coast of present-day Washington and Oregon into the interior. Many infectious diseases—including influenza—moved up the Columbia River and its tributaries, killing Indians indiscriminately, and took their toll among many tribes, including Indians living on the banks of the Columbia and Yakima rivers. In 1832 a "great mortality" traveled in the Northwest the cause of which Boyd identifies as pneumonia, but it may have been linked to influenza.[83] The Yakama were not spared infections of influenza, nor was the disease confined to the nineteenth century. In 1918 the Yakama suffered the effects of the Spanish Influenza, a strain of the influenza virus that affected people throughout the world, killing millions. Interestingly, it killed few Yakama infants and children but had a devastating impact on elders of the Nation.[84]

Cancer

The eighth leading cause of death on the Yakama Reservation was cancer (figure 1.2), including all varieties of the disease. According to the Death Certificates, Yakama people died of many types of cancer afflicting the stomach, liver, lungs, cervix, uterus, breasts, bladder, blood, intestines, rectum, pancreas, and other parts of the body. Specifically, Death Certificates reveal several types of cancer that took the lives of Yakama people, including "uterine cancer," "carcinoma of cervix," and "carcinoma of liver."[85] Cancer is a disease usually characterized by malignant cells multiplying and spreading uncontrollably. Cancer can develop in any part of the body and result in a malignant tumor. Cancer can spread from one area to the next, affecting vital organs. It can develop in blood, muscle, liver, lung, bladder, brain, or other parts of the body. It is not always deadly, but cancer treatment during much of the era under discussion was not well developed.

On the Yakama Reservation, cancer contributed to the deaths of a larger number of females (N = 58/71 percent) than males, and females suffered uterine, cervical, stomach, and breast cancer.[86] In recent years, scientists have suggested that cervical cancer, a leading killer of Yakama women, "may result from microbial infections."[87] These forms of cancer were major killers of Yakama women between 1888 and 1964, but neither men nor women suffered severely from lung cancer. Indeed, lung cancer claimed the lives of 2 females and 3 males during this period and the reason is likely the lack of tobacco use among the Yakama prior to World War II. Tobacco was a sacred plant among native peoples of the Columbia Plateau, and although they used it ceremonially, most of them did not use tobacco on a daily basis. While only 5 Yakama died of lung cancer, cancer of all kinds killed 82 (3 percent) of Yakama Indians. Significantly, although cancer was a leading cause of death on the Yakama Reservation, it was not as prevalent as it was among whites, non-whites, or the people of Washington state.[88]

Premature Births

Premature births (figure 3.10) were the ninth leading cause of death on the reservation, and pertained only to fetuses dead before birth. Prematurity is described as the birth of a baby before 37 weeks' gestation. This "cause of death" contributed to the large number of deaths of infants recorded on the Yakama Reservation (N = 64/61 percent), particularly among males who were born prematurely more frequently than females. This same pattern also holds true for stillbirths, which took the lives of more males than females. Stillbirths and premature births account in large part for the high fetal death rate among the Yakama. Physicians and medical officials refer to still birth as intrauterine death of a fetus when the baby is born dead after the twenty-eighth week of pregnancy.

The mother's health is a crucial factor in premature births. including malnutrition, kidney disease, hypertension (high blood pressure), heart disease, and diabetes. Mothers may also be weak and prone to premature births and stillbirths because poor diets were common among mothers on the Yakama Nation in the early twentieth century. Yakama mothers with any of these conditions were more likely to place the fetus in jeopardy and give birth prematurely.[89] Premature births can be caused by spontaneous abortion, incompetent cervix, hydramnios, and premature rupture of membranes. Spontaneous abortion is commonly known as miscarriage, and it occurs when labor begins before the twentieth week of pregnancy. Premature births can occur when the fetus and placenta separate from the uterus, which may be brought on if one of the organs is defective or if the mother falls or is in an accident. In such cases, when the fetus is rejected before the twentieth week of life, it usually dies.[90]

Premature birth can also be caused by an incompetent cervix, a condition in which the cervix dilates early. Most often this occurs after the fourteenth week of pregnancy when the placenta and fetus detach from the inner uterus, causing a miscarriage. The cervix may be weak and unable to remain closed for nine months. In some cases, the cervix opens early, delivering the baby prematurely. This kind of birth may also be caused by hydramnios which is an accumulation of amniotic fluid inside the uterine wall. In most cases, the accumulation of fluid is harmless, but in some cases, the uterus swells with the fluid and labor begins early. Although these cases are rare, they can occur, particularly if the mothers are diabetic, carry two or more fetuses, or suffer from toxemia.

In addition to the causes mentioned above, premature birth can also occur if the membrane surrounding the baby ruptures. This is called "breaking water," and it is always part of the normal birthing process. In order for there to be a delivery, the membranes must burst, but if the membrane breaks early, infection can develop before the baby is delivered. This can endanger the life of the baby and mother. The rupture of the membrane surrounding the baby can lead to premature birth which, like infection, can endanger the baby's life.[91] Any of these causes of premature birth may have contributed to the premature delivery of fetuses on the Yakama Reservation. However, the actual cause of most miscarriages is unknown. On the Yakama Reservation, the descriptions provided in the Death Certificates generally state that the cause of death was "prematurity," "premature development," or "premature birth." In a few descriptive cases, officials wrote that the death of an infant was caused by "immature birth," "hemorrhage premature," "premature with syphilis," "malnutrition and premature birth," and "premature birth sibling of" (indicating the birth of twins).[92]

Although stillbirths (N = 41/39 percent) were not among the ten leading explanations given for deaths on the Yakama Reservation, they were not far below, ranking thirteenth in the accounting for deaths among the general population, and one of the two significant causes of fetal death (figure 3.10). For this reason, it deserves some discussion. Medical professionals refer to stillbirth as intrauterine death of a fetus, and it occurs when a fetus is delivered after the twentieth week of life. A mother suffering from toxemia or diabetes may contribute to the delivery of a stillborn child. Stillbirth can also be caused by a hemorrhage or an abnormality in the fetus.[93] Like premature births, "stillbirths are more common in poor communities, among older women, and when good prenatal and obstetric care are lacking."[94] Fetuses may be severely malformed and their condition may account for some stillbirths. Malnutrition, hypertension, alcoholism, or ante partum hemorrhage in the mother may also produce stillbirths. If a mother's placenta does not function correctly, a baby may be born dead. This is particularly true if the fetus does not receive sufficient oxygen. A mother who is suffering from measles, rubella, herpes, syphilis, malaria, influenza, chickenpox, or other infectious diseases may also deliver a stillborn baby that was, in fact, a victim of the disease.[95] All of these maladies may have caused stillbirths on the Yakama Reservation, although the Death Certificates and hospital records are silent on this point. Some of these conditions could have been prevented through childbirth education, prenatal care, and preventive medicine.

Senility and Old Age

On the other end of the age spectrum, senility (figure 1.2) and old age accounted for the tenth leading cause of death on the Yakama Reservation (N = 57/3 percent), closely followed by strokes and alcohol-related deaths. Today, senility is described as "Changes in mental ability caused by old age."[96] The condition is associated with loss of memory and concentration with the "risk of *dementia*, which affects about one in five of those over 80."[97] In the past, the term senility was used to describe old age, and county and state officials used the term in the Yakama Death Certificates as a generic and common cause of death. In the early Death Certificates, recording officials noted this cause of death by writing that the person had died of "old age," "senility," or "Inanition & debility-senility." Most often, officials designated the cause of death simply by stating that the person had died of senility, but this description is found primarily in those Death Certificates recorded between 1915 and 1932. It is only used twice as a cause of death after 1932. People who died of this cause had likely lost control of their intellectual abilities and some may have suffered from dementia due to Alzheimer's disease. State and county recording agents may have also used the designation of senility if the deceased person was elderly and officials did not know the exact cause of death.[98]

Place of Death

Place of death is a nominal variable, and all deaths that occurred on and off the reservation were coded. Deaths occurring at unknown locations were also coded. Place of death was often designated on the Death Certificates. If reservation Indians died at Fort Simcoe, Toppenish, Harrah, White Swan, or Wapato, they were coded as having died on the reservation. If they died in Yakima City, Sunnyside, Moxee City, Spokane, or Tacoma, they were coded as having died off the reservation. Thus, those who died within the boundary lines of the reservation were coded as having died on the reservation, even though some of these individuals died in close proximity to the reservation and had lived on the reservation. This method of coding was employed in spite of the fact that traditional lands of Yakama Indians included far more territory than was so designated in the Yakama Treaty of 1855 or was recognized by the United States as trust lands of the Yakama Reservation after allotment.[99]

Yakama Reservation boundary lines changed over time and represent an artificial land division imposed on the Yakama Nation by the government. The boundaries are non-traditional to Indian people, but they have been a part of Yakama history and the legal relationship between the Yakama Nation and the United States since the Senate ratified and the President signed the Yakama Treaty in 1859. For the purposes of this study, reservation boundaries during the early twentieth century were used in spite of their shortcomings, simply to examine where deaths occurred. A total of 2,846 (73 percent) deaths occurred on the Yakama Reservation, while 932 (24 percent) deaths took place off the reservation. State officials did not report the place of death of 121 (3 percent) people.

Place of death and tribal affiliation (Yakama or non-Yakama) were examined to determine if Yakama people generally died on their own reservation. Of the 2,846 Indians who died on the reservation, 2,164 (76 percent) were Yakama, 449 (16 percent) were non-Yakama (but most were identified tribally as among the people who were party to the Yakama Treaty of 1855), and 233 (8 percent) were not known. Of the 932 Native Americans who died off the Yakama Reservation, 391 (42 percent) were Yakama, 221 (24 percent) were non-

Yakama, and the tribal identity of 320 (34 percent) were not known. Yakama Indians died more often on their reservation than off the reservation, and this is generally true of non-Yakama who were either visiting or living on the Yakama Reservation at the time of death. Often the non-Yakama were Indians from tribes who were parties to the Yakama Treaty but who had lived on other Northwestern reservations. Sometimes they were Native Americans who had married or were related to a Yakama person. After an evaluation of this data, the author determined it was not sufficiently significant historically to warrant a further examination in the analysis done in this work. While the data was interesting, it revealed little about Yakama deaths over time and little more than that which is mentioned above.

The fact that most deaths of Yakama Indians occurred on the reservation was likely due to the fact that the reservation was the land base and home of most Yakama Indians. In addition, transportation systems were poor during much of the late nineteenth and early twentieth centuries, so many Indians were without motor vehicles. Yakama Indians did not die in truck and automobile accidents to any marked extent until the 1940s when the first major series of fatalities occurred. People sometimes visited reservation border towns to purchase groceries and other goods, but most people lived on the reservation. When individuals became ill, they remained home, particularly Indian people who received some medical care from nurses, doctors, and medicine people on their home reservation. Most important, they had the help of their families and friends on the reservation. Because of racial issues and the lack of money, Indians were less likely to receive medical care off the reservation. Therefore, when individuals became ill, they tended to remain home where they had familial support and some government medical care.

Tribal Affiliation and Enrollment

Two designations were used to describe a person's tribal affiliation, Yakama and non-Yakama. Each native person in the data set was coded as Yakama, non-Yakama, or unknown. At times, the person's tribal affiliation was illegible, unrecorded, or unknown. A person's tribal affiliation was determined by the statement appearing on the Death Certificates regarding race, and recorders nearly always identified a person as Yakama or Indian. Some Death Certificates, particularly the early ones, also provide the person's blood quantum. However, this was the case for the early data only, and the number of cases is insufficient to draw many conclusions. A person's blood quantum was often indicated in that space provided on the Death Certificates for race, and the person recording the death would often write "Yakama, full-blood" or "4/4 Yakama." As previously stated, the Yakama Reservation was and is the home of people from fourteen different tribes and bands. This included people who traditionally spoke various dialects of three different language families. Thus, the Yakama were and are a confederation of tribes and bands, not a homogeneous group. The Yakama Nation is comprised of several different peoples whom the United States forced onto a single land base under the terms of the Yakama Treaty of 1855.[100]

In addition, the Yakama and their neighbors commonly married Indians outside their group, and this tradition continued after the government established the reservation. Thus, people from several other tribes—Umatilla, Cayuse, Wanapum, Entiat, Nez Perce, Quinault, Nisqually, Spokane, Okanagan, and others—lived on the reservation. The Yakama customarily received guests from many different tribes and bands from Canada and the United States. Some of these people visited the reservation, and some of them lived there for a time. These newcomers onto the Yakama Reservation contributed to the growth in numbers of the Yakama population during the course of the twentieth century. The population grew because of births, as well as because Indians moved off the so-called "public domain"—former Indian lands—onto the reservation. Many diverse Indian people lived and died on the Yakama Reservation, particularly other Pacific Northwest Indians. Most often, recording officials designated a dead person as "Yakama" or "Not Yakama," but at other times, officials recorded the tribe or reservation of the person (see the discussion, below on blood quantum). Of the 3,899 people recorded in the Yakama Death Certificates, 2,568 (66 percent) were Yakama, 681 (18 percent) were non-Yakama, and the identity of 650 (16 percent) Indians was unknown.

On many of the early Death Certificates, the documents had a designation for tribal enrollment. The enrollment of a person did not appear on over two-thirds of the Death Certificates, and the data is incomplete regarding the enrollment status of many people who died on the reservation. If a person was an enrolled member of a tribe, recording officials indicated this on the Death Certificate. The early data indicates whether or not a person was an enrolled member of any tribe, when such information was known. The tribal enrollment of 2,501 (64 percent) of the dead was not known. When enrollment data was cited, a total of 1,396 (36 percent) were enrolled members of a tribe, while only 2 people were not enrolled. Clearly, of those cases that were known, people were enrolled members of a tribe. However, after an evaluation of the data generated regarding the variables of tribal affiliation and tribal enrollment, these variables were incomplete and would not be addressed in this analysis of death.

Ward and Blood Quantum

Ward is a nominal variable, and it is not an important one in this study. If a person was an enrolled member of a tribe that had a legal relationship with the United States government, the Office of Indian Affairs considered that Indian to be a ward or charge of the government. The designation of a person as ward is found only on the early Death Certificates, and this category is not found on over two thirds of the documents. However, the documents from the earlier period indicate that nearly every dead person was a ward, and on those documents, only two individuals (the same two who were recorded as not enrolled) were recorded as not being wards. On the other hand, Death Certificates record a total of 139 (36 percent) people as being wards, while 2,501 (64 percent) are recorded as "unknown" in terms of wardship. These are the same statistics as those found for tribal enrollment, since an enrolled person was considered a ward of the United States. Whether a person was a ward of the government or not had little bearing on this study and is not presented in the analysis of the data.

Blood quantum (figure 3.16) is a nominal variable, and, as nearly all of the population were full-bloods, it is worthy of note. The blood quantum of individuals was generally provided in earlier Death Certificates under the category of race. Sometimes officials recorded that a person was "4/4 Yakama Indian," "3/4 Yak. Ind.," "1/4 Yak. Ind.," "4/4 Idaho Indian," "Chinook Indian," "1/2 Yakama Ind.-1/2 Filipino," or "Unknown degree & kind of Indian."[101] Blood quantum was coded for full-bloods, three-fourth bloods, one-half bloods, one-quarter bloods, and people of unknown blood quantum.

Of the 3,899 Indians analyzed in the data, the blood quantum of 2,640 (68 percent) was provided. Of the latter, 2,213 (84 percent) were full-bloods, 263 (10 percent) were one-half or more but less than full, 164 (6 percent) were quarter-bloods. Thus, the blood quantum of a total of 1,259 (32 percent) Yakama was unknown. Unfortunately, the low number of mixed-bloods makes it difficult to assess the differences between the groups. Although it is generally held that full-bloods suffered more from contagious diseases than did mixed-bloods, because they lacked natural biological immunities to disease introduced by non-Indians, it is difficult to compare the groups because of the small number of mixed-bloods represented in the death population of Yakama. The author expected to find full-bloods dying more often in the population than mixed-bloods. Between 1888 and 1964, this was the case, but full-bloods made up 84 percent of the death population, while mixed-bloods made up a mere 16 percent. Any discussion of the role of blood quantum, cause of death, and numbers of deaths, must take into consideration the fact that there were few mixed-bloods in the death population of the Yakama during these seventy-six years. A brief discussion of blood quantum in relation to the ten leading causes of death is addressed in the Appendix.

Notes

1. Trafzer and Scheuerman, *Renegade Tribe*, 46, 58, 95, 104, 122, 126–131, 135, 137, 140–42.

2. Yakama Death Certificates, NA, PNWR, RG 75.

3. For a thorough examination of the historical literature of the Yakama and other Sahaptin-speaking Indians of the Northwest, see Clifford E. Trafzer, *Yakima, Palouse, Cayuse, Umatilla, Walla Walla, and Wanapum Indians: An Historical Bibliography* (Metuchen, New Jersey: The Scarecrow Press, 1991).

4. Omran, "Epidemiologic Transition in the United States," 16–18.

5. The finest scholarly work on the topic is Boyd, "Introduction of Infectious Diseases Among the Indians of the Pacific Northwest, 1774–1874, " 99–141.

6. Robert H. Ruby and John A. Brown, *Indians of the Pacific Northwest: A History* (Norman: University of Oklahoma Press, 1981), 171–73, 227–30.

7. "Tuberculosis Among North American Indians," *Report of a Committee of the National Tuberculosis Association Appointed on October 28, 1921, on Tuberculosis Among the North American Indians*, 6th Cong., 4th Sess. (Washington, D.C.: Government Printing Office, 1923), 53–72. Yakama Death Certificates are not complete prior to 1924, nor for the number of Yakama deaths resulting from tuberculosis for the years from 1888 to 1923.

8. Popkin, "Nutritional Patterns and Transitions," 138–45.

9. Samuel H. Preston and Michael R. Haines, *Fatal Years: Child Mortality in Late Nineteenth-Century America* (Princeton, New Jersey: Princeton University Press, 1991), 171; George Alter, "Infant and Child Mortality in the United States," paper prepared for "La mortalité des enfants dans le passé," *International Union for the Scientific Study of Population*, University of Montreal (7–9 October 1992): 6–7.

10. Preston and Haines, *Fatal Years*, xix.

11. Much more will be known about the pre-reservation period after the author completes his next study of the Yakama Indian Census from 1885 to 1930. This analysis will help test the hypothesis offered by historians that the reservation system was detrimental to the health of native people who died in large numbers once they were forced onto the reservation.

12. John R. Weeks to Clifford E. Trafzer, 15 June 1994, author's collection.

13. Ibid.

14. Edward D. Castillo, "The Impact of Euro-American Exploration and Settlement," *California*, edited by Robert F. Heizer (Washington, D.C.: Smithsonian Institution Press, 1978), 118, 123, 124; Keith H. Basso, "Western Apache," and Robert L. Bergman, "Navajo Health Services and Projects," *Southwest*, edited by Alfonso Ortiz (Washington, D.C.: Smithsonian Institution Press, 1983), 482-83, 672-77; Clifford E. Trafzer and Richard D. Scheuerman, *Chief Joseph's Allies* (Newcastle: Sierra Oaks Publishing Company, 1992), 83-87; Russell Thornton, *American Indian Holocaust and Survival: A Population History Since 1492* (Norman: University of Oklahoma Press, 1987), 99-104, 125-27.

15. *Puyallup Tribe v. Department of Game*, Supreme Court of the United States, 1968, 391, United States 392, 88 Supreme Court 1725, 20 L. Ed. 2nd 689, in David H. Getches and Charles F. Wilkinson, *Federal Indian Law* (St. Paul, Minnesota: West Publishing Co., 1986), 734-40. The law discussed in this case is applied to the Yakama and appeared in the 1969 case, *Sohappy v. Smith*, and the 1974 case, *United States v. Washington*.

16. Kappler, *Indian Law*, 698-702; Documents Relating to Negotiations of Ratified and Unratified Treaties of the United States, NA, RG 75, Microfilm T494, Reel 5. During the treaty negotiations at the Walla Walla Council, Stevens' specifically guaranteed the Yakama and others the continued right to fish, hunt, and gather wherever they had done so in the past, both on and off the reservation.

17. Trafzer and Beach, "Smohalla, the Washani, and Religion as a Factor in Northwestern Indian History," 73, 75-77. Although Plateau Indians had acquired seeds from Hudson Bay Company traders and had planted gardens, they continued to maintain their traditional economic life. During the early reservation era, some

of the people ranched and farmed, but most continued traditional seasonal rounds. But with the destruction of the root grounds, salmon, and game, Indians turned to ranching and farming. See Schuster, "Yakima Indian Traditionalism," 204, 238, 262. For destruction of salmon through irrigation projects, see Yakima Tribal Council, *The Yakimas: Treaty Centennial, 1855–1955* (Yakima, Washington: Republic Press, 1955), 36, 48. The dams in the Northwest also destroyed the salmon runs. See these general studies on dams located on the Columbia River and its tributaries: United States Department of the Army, *Review Report on Columbia River and Tributaries*, Corps of Engineers, North Pacific Division, 1 October 1948; United States Department of Interior, "The Columbia River," H. Exec. Doc. 473, 81st Cong., 2d Sess. 1950; Bureau of Indian Affairs, *Report on the Source, Nature and Extent of the Fishing, Hunting and Miscellaneous Related Rights of Certain Tribes in Washington and Oregon...* (Los Angeles: Office of Indian Affairs, Division of Forestry and Grazing, 1942); and T. W. Mermel, ed. and comp., *Register of Dams in the United States: Completed, Under Construction and Proposed* (New York: McGraw Hill, 1958).

18. Schuster, *The Yakima*, 29–30.

19. L. V. McWhorter, *The Crime Against the Yakima* (North Yakima, Washington: Republic Press, 1913). McWhorter reported that the Yakama lived in one- or two-room shacks with lean-to kitchens. Also see Schuster, "Yakima Indian Traditionalism," 68–87.

20. Omran, "Epidemiologic Transition in the United States," 8, 9, 18.

21. Schuster, "Yakima Indian Traditionalism," 165–76.

22. Trafzer and Scheuerman, *Renegade Tribe*, 26; S. F. Cook, "The Epidemic of 1830–33 in California and Oregon," *University of California Publications in Archaeology and Ethnology* 43 (1955): 303–26; Thornton, *American Indian Holocaust*, 99.

23. Yakama Death Certificates, NA, PNWR, RG 75. Many unknown cases can be cited, including 4537, 4540, 4541, 4542, 4543, 4552, 4558. The author chose not to disclose the name of any person found on the Death Certificates in order to protect the privacy of Yakama families. Some of the data from the *Annual Reports of the Commissioners of Indian Affairs* are addressed in part four of this work. Some of the difficulties in using these statistics are illustrated in the *Annual Reports of the Commissioner of Indian Affairs*

for 1888, 1889, 1890, 1895, and 1900. In 1888, the document mentions 1 scrofula death and 36 cases among the Yakama (234), but the report of 1889 contains no statistical information on deaths among the Yakama, stating only that "Srcofula and consumption are prevailing ailments" (292). In 1890, the report indicates that the Yakama are suffering with 44 cases of tuberculosis and 41 cases of scrofula (492). In 1895, no mention is made of deaths resulting from any particular causes, although the document notes that there had been 37 births and 29 deaths that year (322). And in 1900, the report deals with an outbreak of smallpox but does not mention tuberculosis or any other disease (400). Sometimes the information on deaths on the Yakama Reservation is helpful, but it is erratic and not consistent.

24. Diane T. Putney, "Robert Grosvenor Valentine, 1909-1912," in Robert M. Kvasnicka and Herman J. Viola, eds., *The Commissioners of Indian Affairs* (Lincoln: University of Nebraska Press, 1979), 233-42. Putney has also written an outstanding scholarly work on Indian health from 1900 to 1930. See Diane T. Putney, "Fighting the Scourge: American Indian Morbidity and Federal Policy, 1897-1928" (Ph. D. dissertation, Marquette University, 1980). A more recent examination of Valentine and other commissioners who dealt with Indian health is found in Todd Benson, "Race, Health, and Power: The Federal Government and American Indian Health, 1909-1955" (Ph. D. dissertation, Stanford University Press, 1993), 1-41.

25. Schuster, "Yakima Indian Traditionalism," 80-83. Allotment of the Yakama Reservation ended in 1914 with 4,506 Yakama people securing for themselves 440,000 acres of individual allotments and 780,000 of tribally owned land. In 1992, the Yakama owned 253,280 acres of the original 440,000 acres, and most of the best farmland with water had been purchased by non-Indians.

26. Scholars should take note of the excellent work recently completed by Todd Benson of Stanford University on the health care of Native Americans during the early twentieth century before the Public Health Service took over Indian health care. Benson has conducted the most in-depth research on the topic. See Benson, "Race, Health, and Power: The Federal Government and American Indian Health, 1909-1955."

27. "Tuberculosis Among North American Indians," 35.

28. *Annual Report of the Commissioner of Indian Affairs, 1888*, 234 and *1889*, 292.

29. *Annual Report of the Commissioner of Indian Affairs, 1890*, 492.

30. "Tuberculosis Among North American Indians," 23, 35–38.

31. Ibid., 38.

32. Ibid., 53, 56, 58, 60, 63, 65, 67, 70, 72.

33. Lawrence C. Kelly, "Charles Henry Burke, 1921–29" and "Charles James Rhoads, 1929–33," and Kenneth R. Philp, "John Collier, 1933–45," in Kvasnicka and Viola, *The Commissioners of Indian Affairs*, 253, 255, 268, 277. The author will provide further analysis of crude death rates, but the evidence is overwhelming that the agents on the Yakama Reservation did not record any infant deaths. In a comparison of death rates, the rates on the reservation are markedly lower than those for the United States as per 1,000 in the population. For example, in 1920, the United States crude death rate was 10, with 1 on the Yakama Reservation. However, birth records are available for the Yakama from 1926 through 1931, and an infant mortality rate is calculated in the analysis which demonstrates the high rate of infant mortality.

34. Lewis Meriam, *The Problem of Indian Administration* (New York: The Johnson Reprint Corp., 1971), 170–82.

35. Ibid., 189.

36. Ibid.

37. Ibid.

38. Ibid., 266.

39. Ibid.

40. Ibid.

41. De Lien and Hadley, "How to Recognize an Indian Health Problem," 33.

42. Ibid.

43. Ibid.

44. Yakama Indian Census, 1885–1931, PNWR, NA, RG 75, Seattle, Washington.

45. Yakama Death Certificates, 1888 to 1910, NA, PNWR, RG 75.

46. No attempt is made to compare the Death Certificates of the Yakama Reservation with any other reservation since no data base exists to do so, except the original Death Certificates or Registers for other reservations in the National Archives. The author plans to collect and analyze some of these documents in the future and use them to compare with the Yakama data.

47. René and Jean Dubos, *The White Plague: Tuberculosis, Man, and Society* (New Brunswick: Rutgers University Press, [1952] 1987), 185–87.

48. Meriam, *The Problem of Indian Affairs*, 189–345; Kenneth R. Philp, *John Collier's Crusade for Indian Reform, 1920–1954* (Tucson: University of Arizona Press, 1977), 114, 126–27, 130, 134.

49. Preston and Haines, *Fatal Years*, xxi; Benson, "Race, Health, and Power," 238–323.

50. Hunn to Trafzer, 18 May 1994.

51. Ibid.

52. Trafzer and Scheuerman, *Renegade Tribe*, 25–26, Robert H. Ruby and John A. Brown, *The Cayuse Indians* (Norman: University of Oklahoma Press, 1972), 103–8; Clifford E. Trafzer, *The Chinook* (New York: Chelsea House Publishers, 1990), 34–35; Boyd, "The Introduction of Infectious Diseases Among the Indians of the Pacific Northwest, 1774–1874," 81–90, 99–100, 112–45, and 338–50. Also see Hunn, *Nch'i–Wana*, 27–32, 241.

53. Omran, "Epidemiologic Transition in the United States," 16.

54. Yakama Death Certificates, NA, PNWR, RG 75, Cases 4795, 462, 2768, 1203, 206, 2958, 489, 696, 3462, 3565.

55. For a historical perspective of the importance of disease, see Alfred W. Crosby, *The Columbian Exchange: The Biological and Cultural Consequences of 1492* (Westport: Greenwood Publishing Co., 1972); Frederick Fox Cartwright, *Disease and History* (London: Hart–Davis, 1972); Howard Simpson, *Invisible Armies* (Indianapolis: Bobbs-Merrill, 1980); William H. McNeill, *Plagues and Peoples* (New York: Doubleday, 1976); and Ann F. Ramenofsky, *Vectors of Death* (Albuquerque: University of New Mexico Press, 1987).

56. For a general work on methods, see Colin Newell, *Methods and Models in Demography* (London: Belhaven Press, 1988). Also, for

specifics on crude death rates and infant mortality, see John R. Weeks, *Population: An Introduction to Concepts and Issues* (Belmont, California: Wadsworth, 1992), 170-71, 177-82; Henry S. Shryock, Jacob S. Siegel, and Associates, *The Methods and Materials of Demography* (San Diego: Academic Press, 1976), 224-25, 237-38.

57. Dubos and Dubos, *The White Plague*, xix.

58. Ibid., 4-10; F. B. Smith, *The Retreat of Tuberculosis, 1850-1950* (London: Croom Helm, 1988), 2-5; Richard Harrison Shryock, *National Tuberculosis Association, 1904-1954* (New York: National Tuberculosis Association, 1957), 2-7, 43-44, 49-53, 59-71, 234-36.

59. Dubos and Dubos, *The White Plague*, 5-6.

60. Ibid., Case 1160; Jeffrey R. M. Kunz and Asher J. Finkel, *The American Medical Association Family Medical Guide* (New York: Random House, 1987), 574, 719, 748; Wesley W. Spink, *Infectious Diseases: Prevention and Treatment in Nineteenth and Twentieth Centuries* (Minneapolis: University of Minnesota Press, 1978), 209-12, 220-21, 224; Ales Hrdlicka, "Tuberculosis Among Certain Indian Tribes in the United States," *Annual Report of the Bureau of American Ethnography* 42 (Washington, D.C.: Smithsonian Institution, 1909), 32-33; Frank McFarlan Burnet and David O. White, *Natural History of Infectious Diseases* (Cambridge: Cambridge University Press, 1972), 213-24; Jay Arthur Meyers, *Captain of All These Men of Death* (St. Louis, Missouri: Warren H. Green, 1977), 73-83, 142-58; Selman A. Waksman, *The Conquest of Tuberculosis* (Berkeley: University of California Press, 1964), 24, 204-8. The most penetrating and significant work on the subject in recent years is Barbara Bates, *Bargaining for Life: A Social History of Tuberculosis, 1876-1938* (Philadelphia: University of Pennsylvania Press, 1992).

61. "Tuberculosis Among North American Indians," 53-72.

62. Dubos and Dubos, *The White Plague*, 187.

63. "Tuberculosis," *Med Facts* (Denver: National Jewish Center for Immunology and Respiratory Medicine, 1987), 1.

64. Yakama Death Certificates, NA, PNWR, RG 75, Cases 179, 202, 701, 2837, 3031.

65. Charles B. Clayman, ed., *The American Medical Association Encyclopedia of Medicine* (New York: Random House, 1989): 803.

66. Spink, *Infectious Diseases*, 209–12; Burnet and White, *Natural History of Infectious Diseases*, 32–43, 52–69; Andrew B. Christie, *Infectious Diseases: Epidemiology and Clinical Practice* (Edinburgh and London: E. and S. Livingstone, 1969), 269–99; and Kunz and Finkel, *Family Medical Guide*, 365, 6–95. For general medical studies, specifically on pneumonia, see William S. Lynn, ed., *Inflammatory Cells and Lung Disease* (Boca Raton, Florida.: CRC Press, 1983); James E. Pennington, ed., *Respiratory Infections: Diagnosis and Management* (New York: Raven Press, 1983); Selwyn DeWitt Collins and Josephine Lehmann, *Excess Deaths from Influenza and Pneumonia and from Important Chronic Diseases During Epidemic Periods, 1918–1951* (Washington, D.C., Public Health Service, 1953).

67. Clayman, ed., *Encyclopedia of Medicine*, 803.

68. Oral discussion, 17 February 1995, University of California, Berkeley.

69. Yakama Death Certificates, NA, PNWR, RG 75, Cases 2445, 231, 476, 697.

70. Popkin, "Nutritional Patterns and Transitions," 138–46.

71. Omran, "Epidemiologic Transition in the United States," 17.

72. Kunz and Finkle, *Family Medical Guide*, 380–86.

73. Ibid., 388, 640.

74. Ibid., 671–72.

75. Yakama Death Certificates, NA, PNWR, RG 75, Cases 118, 49, 588, 3203, 3402, 3789, 3835, 2933.

76. Ibid., Cases 70, 336, 94, 597, 9930, 2387, 2839, 3486, 3872, 3494.

77. Kunz and Finkle, *Family Medical Guide*, 467, 664, 702; Christie, *Infectious Diseases*, 122–67; Spink, *Infectious Diseases*, 246–47; Burnet and White, *Natural History of Infectious Diseases*, 70–87. For general medical works on gastrointestinal disorders, see Marvin H. Sleisenger and John S. Fordtran, eds., *Gastrointestinal Disease* (Philadelphia: W. B. Saunders, 1989); Emanuel Lebenthan, ed., *Textbook of Gastroenterology and Nutrition in Infancy* (New York: Raven Press, 1981); and S. C. Truelove, *Diseases of the Digestive System* (Oxford: Blackwell Scientific Publications, 1972).

Another form of gastrointestinal disorder is caused by a viral infection from food and liquid, although this is rare.

78. Yakama Death Certificates, NA, PNWR, RG 75, Cases 478, 611, 865, 1293, 2427, 2696, 4510.

79. Ibid., Cases 3845, 2401, 2971, 3565, 3759, 774, 2927, 4132, 4193, 4522. Automobile accidents caused several deaths among Yakama who were over the age of six. If a person was driving a car and was hit and killed by a train, the death was coded as an automobile accident. If a person was intoxicated and killed in an automobile accident, the death was coded automobile accident. Overall deaths by this cause ranked sixth during the seventy-six year period from 1888 to 1964.

80. Kunz and Finkle, *Family Medical Guide*, 365, 570-71.

81. Yakama Death Certificates, NA, PNWR, RG 75, Cases 9245, 247, 2402, 3984, 3989, 246, 338, 1145, 1287.

82. Boyd, "The Introduction of Infectious Diseases Among the Indians of the Pacific Northwest, 1774-1874," 113-18.

83. Ibid., 346-47.

84. Trafzer, *The Chinook*, 34-35.

85. Yakama Death Certificates, NA, PNWR, RG 75, Cases 536, 605, 1236, 2429, 3189, 3463, 3510, 3584, 3791, 3847, 4001, 4517, 4417.

86. According to Brad Richie, M.D., and Professor James Sandos, University of Redlands, doctors could not distinguish between uterine and cervical cancers without conducting autopsies. It is unlikely that many autopsies, if any, were performed on these women. Sandos suggested that the two types of cancer would be more properly labeled venereal cancer. Oral interviews by the author with Richie and Sandos, 1995.

87. F. Xavier Bosch, et al. "Male Sexual Behavior and Human Papilloma-Virus DNA: Key Risk Factors for Cervical Cancer in Spain," *Journal of the National Cancer Institute* 88 (1996): 1060-1075. "New, Reemerging, and Drug Resistant Infections," *Home Page* (Atlanta: National Center for Infectious Diseases, 1996), 1.

88. Kunz and Finkle, *Family Medical Guide*, 47, 711.

89. Clayman, ed., *Encyclopedia of Medicine*, 817.

90. Kunz and Finkle, *Family Medical Guide*, 643-48; Wenda R. Trevathan, *Human Birth: An Evolutionary Perspective* (New York:

Aldine de Gruyter, 1987), 12, 21, 67, 93, 98, 119, 124–25, 141–42, 199, 228. For medical studies on premature births, see Beryl Dorothy Corner, *Prematurity: The Diagnosis, Care and Disorders of the Premature Infant* (London: Cassell, 1960); Julius H. Hess and Evelyn C. Lundeen, *The Premature Infant* (Philadelphia: Lippincott, 1949); and Evelyn C. Lundeen and Ralph H. Kunstadter, *Care of the Premature Infant* (Philadelphia: Lippincott, 1958). Most of the medical works on premature births discuss the medical problems of dealing with the child that survives, and they do not analyze the issue of high infant mortality resulting from premature births. The twentieth week is counted from the first day of the mother's last period.

91. Kunz and Finkle, *Family Medical Guide*, 643–48.

92. Yakama Death Certificates, NA, PNWR, RG 75, Cases 4179, 4165, 4384, 878, 699, 3206, 4381, 2377, 2878.

93. Trevathan, *Human Birth*, 11–12, 21, 75, 105, 142; Kunz and Finkle, *Family Medical Guide*, 647.

94. Clayman, ed., *Encyclopedia of Medicine*, 941.

95. Ibid.

96. Ibid., 891.

97. Ibid.

98. Yakama Death Certificates, NA, PNWR, RG 75, Cases 120, 4314; Kunz and Finkle, *Family Medical Guide*, 742.

99. Kappler, *Indian Law*, 698–702.

100. Ruby and Brown, *A Guide to the Indian Tribes of the Pacific Northwest*, 58–62.

101. Yakama Death Certificates, NA, PNWR, RG 75, Cases 3181, 3184, 3190, 3188, 3308, 3271, 3218, 3186.

PART FOUR

COMPARISON OF YAKAMA DEATH RATES WITH OTHER POPULATIONS

Over half of the deaths on the Yakama Reservation between 1888 and 1964 resulted from three major causes, namely tuberculosis, pneumonia, and heart disease (figure 1.2). Comparisons made here in relation to deaths from these diseases are drawn from Yakama Death Certificates which contain clinical, not medical, explanations of death. Unfortunately, the data from the Yakama Death Certificates during the years from 1888 to 1923 are poor and will generally not be used for comparing crude Yakama death rates with the general population of Washington, the African American population, or white population of the United States. A comparative analysis of crude death rates will be offered of data from Yakama Death Certificates primarily for those years from 1924 to 1964, a forty-year period with rich data dealing with Yakama Indian mortality. Some comparisons are given at ten-year intervals from 1930 to 1960, provided that data was available to offer such comparisons. Comparisons of Yakama, African Americans, and whites in the United States are provided in relationship to the ten most frequent causes of death within the general Native American population of the Yakama Reservation.

In order to convey the importance of the 619 (28 percent) deaths from tuberculosis on the Yakama reservation (figures 1.2, 1.4), the study offers comparisons of crude death rates among the Yakama and other populations of the United States.[1] Although these comparisons are between a small population, with relatively few deaths in any one year, and much larger populations, the comparisons are instructive (figures 4.1, 4.2, 4.3). Comparisons of crude death rates are provided per 100,000 in the population for reasons of consistency, because data provided by the federal government is offered per 100,000 in the population.

Tuberculosis

In 1930, the year in which some of the best data is available for the Yakama Reservation, the crude death rate per 100,000 in the population among Yakama people for tuberculosis was 1428. The crude death rate per 100,000 in the population resulting from tuberculosis among African Americans was 192, and in the same year among whites it was 58. The crude death rate per 100,000 people in the population for tuberculosis among the general population of the United States in 1930 was 71 (figure 4.4). Without question, the crude death rate resulting from tuberculosis among Yakama people in 1930 was much higher than other populations.

Several factors contributed to the extraordinarily high crude death rate. The Yakama suffered from tuberculosis in epidemic proportions in the 1920s and 1930s (and perhaps earlier, but Yakama death data is not available to offer such comparisons), and health officials working on the reservation did not have sufficient funding or staff to combat the disease. Agency officials recorded cases of tuberculosis on the reservation in the 1890s and 1910s but provided few statistics regarding death from the disease. Moreover, although the Yakama Agency and Office of Indian Affairs attempted to curb tuberculosis by educating people about the disease, the educational endeavor was not wide-ranging or thorough. As described earlier, Agent Carr tried to instruct Yakama women about sanitation and the spread of disease among infants and children, but his effort in 1917 barely addressed the large problems found in the reservation. Furthermore, Carr tried in vain to have the Office of Indian Affairs build a hospital on the Yakama Reservation, an endeavor that was not begun until 1928.[2]

Tuberculosis is influenced by many factors. What is more, "any human being can become tuberculous if he is exposed to heavy infection while in a state of physiological misery."[3] In eighteenth- and nineteenth-century America, many people believed that tuberculosis was hereditary, but this theory was put to rest by Robert Koch in 1882 when he discovered tubercle bacilli.[4] Although Koch made the discovery, it would take years for some scientists, medical doctors, and nurses to believe that microorganisms caused such a deadly disease. However, the scientific and medical communities after 1882 learned that tubercle bacilli are usually inhaled into the air sacs of the lungs "in droplets of sputum or in particles of dust." The intestines can also become the primary site of infection if food is ingested that is contaminated with tuberculosis. The bacilli are often transported into "the lymph channels to the nearest lymph nodes and multiply there also."[5] Tuberculosis of the lymph nodes is called scrofula, and this manifestation of the disease was particularly acute in the neck of victims.[6] The disease traveled easily in the blood stream, moving from one part of the body to another. Scofula often caused open wounds that oozed blood and pus. Yakama people with this form of tuberculosis used bandages to cover the wounds, and the disease could be spread to those people handling bandages. Tuberculosis was and is a complex and unpredictable disease that was very difficult to detect until it was into its advance stages.[7] Moreover, the best way to detect the disease was through X-rays which were not developed until 1895 and not used on the reservation until the 1930s.[8]

Tuberculosis was caused by exposure to tubercle bacilli, but the course of the disease was influenced by environmental and other factors such as food, housing, fatigue, public health, and mental health.[9] "It is just as important to know what is in a man's head," wrote William Osler, "as what is in his chest."[10] Indeed, many scholars have pointed out the relationship between one's state of mind and one's susceptibility to disease. In their famous study, *The White Plague: Tuberculosis, Man, and*

Society, René and Jean Dubos assert that among the Sioux in 1880, there was "No obvious evidence of tuberculosis . . . at the time that they were compelled to move into barracks in the prison camp; but soon deaths, due to the disease in its most acute form, began to occur." The authors also note the trend among Native Americans to contract tuberculosis in epidemic proportions within the first three decades of their forced re-movals to reservations where they had "to abandon their free way of life."[11]

What was true of the Sioux was true of Chiracahua Apaches under Geronimo who were forced into imprisonment in Florida and Alabama. And what was true of the Apache was true of the Yakama and other free bands of Plateau Indians forced onto the reservation in the late nineteenth century. In his path-breaking study of infectious diseases among Northwestern Indians, Robert Boyd deals with many infectious diseases, including influenza, pneumonia, smallpox, measles, typhus, typhoid, whooping cough, dysentery, but little mention is made regard-ing tuberculosis among Plateau Indians from 1774 to 1874, although it is known to have been present on the Plateau before reaching epidemic proportions in the early twentieth century.[12] Indians had little knowledge about how to deal with infectious diseases, and this is a major reason tuberculosis and other diseases spread within the population. The significance of public health, isolation, sanitation, and general knowledge about how to deal with disease became well known in the general population of the United States in the early twentieth century. But Indians living on reservations and speaking a plethora of languages, lacked the know-how.[13]

Indians also suffered from the destruction of native foods and an absence of nutrition derived from them. The importance of diet as a factor in tuberculosis has not been overlooked at least by some scholars, but, too often ignored or underrated is the fact that the Yakama experienced mortality rates from tuberculosis as a result of factors relating to government Indian policies and the reservation system. Living in poverty and within close proximity to neighbors and mobile non-Indian populations off the reservation, including merchants and rail-men, the Yakama contracted infections, which spread rapidly throughout the reservation. Ironically, they may well have become infected through individuals with tuberculosis from the eastern parts of the country traveling to and through the region seeking rest, relaxation, and clear air in the great American West. Several environmental conditions influenced the spread of tubercular infection on the Yakama Reservation, particularly after 1890.[14]

During the first three decades of the twentieth century, the Yakama lived in poverty with their lives generally restricted to lands lying within the boundaries of the reservation where white farming and ranching destroyed native fruits and vegetables. Depletion of native food resources occurred because non-Indians resettled former Yakama lands and purchased reservation lands after they were allotted by the government. White ranchers and farmers introduced plows, horses, hogs, sheep, and cattle that changed the environment by destroying plant and animal habitats. Although some Yakama Indians farmed and ranched for a portion of their livelihood, many Yakama also hunted, fished, and gathered on and off the reservation during the early years of the twentieth century. However, during the course of the twentieth century, natural food sources dwindled as whites controlled more and more lands on and off the Yakama Reservation. The importance of diet is recognized today as an essential element of Indian health, and the Indian Health Service offers several nutritional and dietetic programs to educate native peoples about food and health.[15] Changes in food sources altered the Yakama diet that was once high in fruits, vegetables, game, and fish.[16] As the government confined people to the reservation, Indians ate more processed foods, particularly those high in carbohydrates.[17] This change of diet was detrimental to the people, weakening their bodies and offering new hosts to disease. The change in diet was accompanied by a change in housing and the seasonal movement of people from root grounds to fishing areas to hunting sites to permanent villages along the rivers. The disruption of their way of life significantly altered the health of the Yakama and other Indians of the region.

Food and housing changes were important in the emergence, spread, and continuance of tuberculosis on the reservation. The disease spread because families no longer moved about, living in mat lodges and tipis, all the while policing their living areas. Permanent shack homes, unventilated and unsanitary, contributed to the spread of tuberculosis and other diseases. Families and agency officials did not isolate patients or teach preventive measures which could have helped control the spread of tuberculosis. Moreover, educational programs might have pointed out that tuberculosis was spread through coughing, spitting, and touching, as well as through the sharing of cups, glasses, knives, forks, spoons, blankets, pipes, quilts, and clothing that had been contaminated with sputum filled with tubercle bacilli. Yakama people had little or no knowledge about sanitizing such material items before using them, and they knew little about the emerging concern for public health. Yakama people, agency officials, and the medical staff on the reservation were unable to prevent the tuberculosis epidemic that ravaged the Yakama Reservation during the first half of the twentieth century for several reasons, including those mentioned above.[18]

In 1940, tuberculosis ranked first as the leading cause of death on the Yakama Reservation and accounted for 26 percent of all deaths that year (figure 4.4). The crude death rate per 100,000 caused by tuberculosis in the Yakama population was 868. The death rate per 100,000 in the population during the same year was 128 among African Americans, 37 among whites, and 46 in the general population of the United States. Thus, the crude death rate among Yakama in 1940 due to tuberculosis was much higher than the crude death rate among other peoples of the United States. Although antibiotics had been in use for over a decade, effective antibiotic treatment for tuberculosis was not refined until the 1950s. Rates for deaths caused by tuberculosis on the Yakama Reservation remained extremely high during the 1930s, and the crude death rate in 1940 mirrored a continuing health problem on the reservation. Yakama Indians were not alone in the experience of a tuberculosis epidemic, and, by the 1930s, bureaucrats working for the United States government could not ignore the alarming number of deaths caused by tuberculosis among Native Americans.

The large number of deaths resulting from tuberculosis on the Yakama and other reservations during the 1920s and 1930s created a demand among reformers and health officials to conquer the disease among American Indians. The result was a concerted effort to eradicate tuberculosis among Native Americans during the 1940s through improved public health, sanitation, sanitoria, diet, and housing. Because of this health initiative during the Indian New Deal era, the health division of the

Office of Indian Affairs, with the help of the Public Health Service, tried to control the spread of tuberculosis within native populations of the United States. Moreover, Indian health officials were aided by the ebb and flow of the disease. "Tuberculosis has waxed and waned several times in the course of human history," according to the Dubos.[19] It is possible that the theory of epidemic waves influenced the radical decline of deaths from tuberculosis on the Yakama Reservation during the 1940s. As a result of several factors, only 3 Indians died of tuberculosis on the Reservation in 1950, a remarkable decline from previous years, creating a crude death rate of 76 per 100,000 in the population (compared to a crude death rate of 868 in 1940). Indeed, between 1950 and 1964, only 13 Yakama died of tuberculosis, indicating sustained declines in the number of deaths caused by this dangerous disease. In 1960, although a few cases of tuberculosis still existed, not one Yakama person died of the disease. By comparison, in 1960 the crude death rate per 100,000 in the population for deaths resulting from tuber- culosis among African Americans was 13 and among white Americans, 5. The national effort to address tuberculosis among the Native American population through public health, diet, antibiotics, and housing was evident in these declining death rates, particularly among the Yakama.[20]

The fact that Yakama people and African Americans suffered higher crude tuberculosis death rates than whites in the United States in 1930 and 1940 was, in part, the result of substandard housing, the lack of public health, poor medical care, and inadequate diets. The disease had ravaged the Yakama popula- tion because of the lack of knowledge about the disease, and about preventive measures that would have led them to quaran- tine victims. Although African Americans, whites, and others within the general population of the United States had some knowledge of how tuberculosis was contracted and treated, most Indians had little knowledge of tuberculosis or how to treat it. Many Yakama did not speak or read English or had minimal ability with the language, making it difficult for them to receive health information in English. Furthermore, there were few communication systems that targeted the Yakama Indian population with newspapers, radio broadcasts, flyers, pamphlets, or general information.[21] Finally, during the early part of the twentieth century, the Yakama did not immediately recognize symptoms of the disease. This was the case in many Native American populations. During the era from 1888 to 1964, tuberculosis was the foremost cause of death among Yakama Indians, but it was particularly virulent from the 1920s to the 1940s.[22]

Pneumonia

Between 1888 and 1964, pneumonia took the lives of 566 (26 percent) Yakama people. It was a major killer of Yakama adults and children alike, and crude death rates resulting from pneumonia for Yakama people were many times that of African Americans, white Americans, and the general public of the United States in 1930, 1940, 1950, and 1960 (figure 4.4). Indeed, inflammation of the lungs was a common respiratory condition of the Yakama—children and adults alike—because bacilli and viruses thrived on the host population. Like tuberculosis, pneumonia was prevalent because of the lack of public health, sanitation, housing, and diet. Poverty, too, helped create poor general health of the Yakama Nation. The same conditions that produced to a high rate of death due to tuberculosis and other diseases held true for deaths resulting from pneumonia.

Poverty contributed significantly to diseases of all kinds on the Yakama Reservation, including pneumonia. The reservation was a virtual host for bacilli and viruses. Pneumonia spread because of conditions on the reservation during much of the twentieth century. With their resistances low due to poor diet, unhealthy housing conditions, insufficient medical care, and anomie, the Yakama contracted pneumonia and died. Other diseases, including tuberculosis, influenza, and gastrointestinal disorders, contributed to deaths from pneumonia—weakening patients to such an extent pneumonia killed them. Tuberculosis was so prevalent on the Yakama Reservation that opportunistic bacilli and common viruses infected the lungs and introduced pneumonia into Yakama people. Like tuberculosis, influenza viruses also weakened some individuals, inviting pneumonia to invade a patient's body. Pneumonia killed many people on the Yakama Reservation, particularly children under six years of age, but unlike tuberculosis, it was not eradicated as a major killer after the 1940s. Pneumonia continued to be a significant cause of death on the reservation throughout the early twentieth century until 1964.

In 1930, the death rate of the Yakama per 100,000 in the population as a result of pneumonia was 850. The crude death rate for African Americans was 12 and for whites it was 3.[23] The crude death rate among the Yakama due to pneumonia was incredibly high in comparison to other American populations. Although the crude death rates resulting from pneumonia declined in all four of the populations by 1940, the disease continued to kill many people in the country, particularly Yakama people who received poor health care and suffered from abject poverty. In 1940, the death rate per 100,000 resulting from pneumonia in the Yakama population was 644. The crude death rate for the same disease among African Americans was 10 and among whites it was 3. Indeed, although the crude death rate caused by pneumonia had declined in the Yakama population in 1940, it was still many times greater than the crude death rate found in other populations of the United States. In 1950, the crude death rate resulting from pneumonia on the reservation had dropped to 126. Significantly, pneumonia continued to plague the Yakama population into the 1960s, a time in which tuberculosis was nearly absent from the reservation. The death rate per 100,000 in the Yakama population resulting from pneumonia in 1960 rose slightly to 133. It was 54 among African Americans and 30 among white Americans. The comparisons are not as dramatic as they were in 1930 and 1940, but pneumonia remained an important cause of death among the Yakama throughout the twentieth century.[24]

In 1940, pneumonia was still the second leading cause of death among the Yakama, and it accounted for 19 percent of all deaths on the reservation that year. In 1950, pneumonia and heart disease were leading causes of death on the Yakama Reservation, each accounting for 17 percent of the deaths that year. In 1960, pneumonia caused 18 percent of the known deaths and ranked third as a leading cause of death on the reservation. During the era from 1888 to 1964, pneumonia was a major cause of death within the Yakama population. This included the years between 1950 and 1964 when tuberculosis declined so dramatically as a cause of death on the Yakama Reservation. Overall pneumonia, remained a significant cause of death among Yakama, African Americans, and whites throughout most of the twentieth century.

Heart Disease

Heart diseases of all kinds contributed to many Yakama deaths (N = 325/15 percent) during the period under discussion, and although heart disease had always been a part of Yakama epidemiological history, it became the foremost cause of death after World War II. Heart disease was the third most significant cause of death on the Yakama Reservation, but its significance as a cause of death increased with time. In 1940, heart disease accounted for 7 percent of all known deaths that year, but by 1960, it accounted for 23 percent of all known deaths on the Yakama Reservation. With the decline of tuberculosis and gastrointestinal disorders as primary causes of death, and with the shift in foods among the Yakama from roots, fish, and game to refined-processed foods, the significance of heart diseases and other man–made degenerative diseases rose. In 1940, the crude death rate of the Yakama per 100,000 resulting from heart disease in the population was 224, and in 1950, the crude death rate had dropped to 126. However, in 1960, the crude death rate among the Yakama due to heart disease had risen to 171, and in that year, heart disease tied miscellaneous accidents as the foremost cause of death on the reservation (figure 4.4). Heart disease grew in importance most likely because of a change in diet, way of life, and increased use of tobacco.

As the years passed during the twentieth century, Yakama lost access to traditional food resources. They were confined to the reservation and not permitted to enter public and private lands—former Yakama lands or lands they had used for generations—to hunt, fish, and gather. Native fish, game, fruits, and vegetables on the Columbia Plateau became depleted in the twentieth century. Hunting and root grounds gave way to farms, ranches, and lumber companies which changed land use, exploiting natural resources and introducing new plants and animals to the earth. Federal and state governments restricted Indian fishing and hunting, and government agencies damned Northwestern rivers, killing thousands of fish each year that once traveled up the Columbia River and its tributaries to spawn. The results were disastrous for Yakama people whose physical, mental, and spiritual health suffered because of the loss of traditional food sources that were closely tied to their religious beliefs. As the Yakama lost their traditional foods, they were forced to seek wage-earning jobs and, with currency, purchase processed foods that were not as nutritious as traditional foods. Furthermore, the new foods eaten by the people were unfamiliar to their bodies and hard to digest, and the Yakama could not take full nutritional value from them. Nontraditional diet harmed the health of Yakama people and dramatically altered traditional life.

Yakama death data for 1900 and 1910 is incomplete, but within the general population of the United States, heart disease was the fourth leading cause of death in 1900 and the foremost cause of death in 1940 and 1960. It was also a leading cause of death among African Americans and whites during the first six decades of the twentieth century. The death rate per 100,000 resulting from heart disease among the Yakama population is not as high as those for other causes of death. The rate of death among Yakama people was about equal to or less than those of other populations in the United States. The Yakama had a slightly higher death rate due to heart disease than African Americans and whites in 1930, but by a very small margin. In 1930, the Yakama crude death rate per 1000,000 in the population was 238, while it was 225 among African Americans and 213 among whites. The Yakama death rate for heart disease in 1930 was less than that of the general population of the United States which had a death rate of 414 per 100,000 in the population.[25]

Heart disease was the third most frequent cause of death on the Yakama Reservation in 1930 and the fourth leading cause of death on the reservation in 1940. In 1950, heart disease as a cause of death became more significant to the Yakama. In that year, heart disease tied pneumonia as the leading cause of death, and in 1960, heart disease became the leading cause of death on the Yakama Reservation, a ranking it shared with miscellaneous accidents. The death rate in the Yakama population resulting from deaths by both heart disease and miscellaneous accidents in 1960 was 171. The increased importance of heart disease as a cause of death on the Yakama Reservation was a result of many factors already mentioned. In the years before 1960, the

Yakama population was harmed more by tuberculosis and pneumonia than by heart disease. With better public and medical health, improved housing and income, and with tuberculosis waning, the number of deaths resulting from tuberculosis and pneumonia decreased while deaths from heart diseases increased.

In addition, heart diseases are linked to the use of tobacco, lack of exercise, depression, and diets high in fats. These factors have contributed greatly to the deaths of thousands of people in the United States, and they influenced the Yakama population during the 1950s after Yakama veterans and defense workers returned to the reservation. The use of tobacco by Yakama people likely changed in the 1940s and 1950s. Tobacco use among traditional Yakama was ceremonial, although the people had known of and used the plant since the time of creation. However, everyday use of tobacco is a fairly recent phenomenon on the Yakama Reservation, a result of contact with non–Indians through advertising and marketing on the reservation and its border towns. During World War II, several Indians from the Yakama Reservation fought in the war or worked in defense industries. Both pursuits brought them into contact with people who used tobacco regularly, and some of these men and women undoubtedly acquired the habit. This, in part, may account for some of the rise in heart disease among the Yakama after 1940.[26]

Traditional Yakama diets had also contributed to the lower number of deaths caused by heart disease, because their diet was once high in vegetables such as camas, bitterroots, kouse, and other nutritious roots. Their diet was high in berries, taken and preserved at different times of the year, and included a good deal of fish, especially salmon, but they also ate such game as deer, rabbit, and bear. However, the bulk of the Yakama diet was fruits and vegetables until the early twentieth century, although they also ate beef and pork on occasion. Thus, the traditional Yakama diet was high in fiber and vitamins and low in fats, especially saturated fats. In the past, men, women, and children had engaged in a good deal of exercise, as they worked and played, often riding horseback or walking to fishing, hunting, root, and berry grounds—on and off the reservation. Their physical activities, particularly moving about, became limited during twentieth century, as white ranchers, farmers, and bureaucrats broke the cycle of Yakama seasonal rounds. Changes in tobacco use, diet, depression, and exercise influenced the rise in heart disease among the people.[27]

As the twentieth century progressed, Yakama diets changed radically from natural foods to processed foods provided by wage earners and government commodities. The change in diet, like that in tobacco use, exercise, and housing, contributed to the ill health of Yakama people. On the other hand, by the 1940s and 1950s, public health education and practices had become more common on the reservation, resulting in the decline of infectious diseases of all kinds. Still, heart disease was an important cause of death throughout the twentieth century, and during the 1950s, the Yakama witnessed a rise in the number of heart-related deaths. For the first time in Yakama history, heart disease, not tuberculosis, became the foremost cause of death. During the decade of the 1950s, the Yakama experienced 82 deaths related to heart disease, and during this ten-year period, they suffered 25 percent of all heart-related deaths of the period from 1888 to 1964. The effects of heart disease mirrored that of the general population of the United States, and this was a significant development in Yakama history.

Miscellaneous Accidents

Miscellaneous accidents unrelated to automobile accidents were the fourth leading cause of death among all Yakama during the era from 1888 to 1964 (N = 145/7 percent). The large number of deaths of Yakama caused by accidents is not uncommon among other populations, but the rate of death by this cause was often many times that of other populations (figure 4.4). For example, in 1930, the crude death rate per 100,000 resulting from miscellaneous accidents was 204 in the Yakama population, while the crude death rate for similar deaths was 64 for African Americans, 53 for whites, and 54 for the general population of the United States. In 1940, the crude death rate per 100,000 resulting from miscellaneous accidents was 112 among the Yakama population, as opposed to 52 among African Americans, 46 among white Americans, and 47 among the general population of the United States. This represented a decline in the Yakama death rate by miscellaneous accidents from that of 1930, but such accidents remained a major cause of death among the people. In 1950, not one Yakama died as a consequence of miscellaneous accidents, but this trend did not continue during the 1950s, as a total of 21 people died of non-automobile related accidents during the decade.[28]

The death rate resulting from miscellaneous accidents increased for the Yakama in 1960. This may have been the result of new technologies and commercial products on the reservation. Miscellaneous accidents were the leading cause of death on the Yakama Reservation in 1960, accounting for 23 percent of all causes of death that year. They shared this dubious distinction with heart disease. In comparison to a Yakama crude death rate per 100,00 of 171, the death rate for this cause of death was 44 among African Americans, 29 among white Americans, and 31 among the general population of the United States. Certainly, miscellaneous accidents were an important cause of death among many diverse populations within the United States during much of the twentieth century, including Yakama Indians who died from train accidents, asphyxiation, rattlesnake bites, drowning, farm equipment accidents, poisonings, and numerous other accidental deaths.[29]

Gastrointestinal Disorders

In marked contrast to other populations within the United States, Yakama Indians suffered severely from gastrointestinal disorders—including diarrhea—during the era from 1888 to 1964 (N = 124/6 percent). Fifth among all causes of death on the Yakama Reservation, gastrointestinal disorders caused numerous deaths before 1950 but few after that year. They were caused by bacilli that infected the stomach and intestines, and particularly affected infants and children. The decline in the number of deaths caused by diseases of the gastrointestinal tract was largely due to advances in public health and sanitation on the Yakama Reservation, including educational programs that informed the population about common bacteria and the simple methods of destroying microorganisms.

In 1930, the death rate among Yakama people per 100,000 in the population as a result of gastrointestinal disorders was 170, and it jumped to 420 in 1940 (figure 4.4). Unfortunately, the data for this cause of death among African Americans and white Americans is combined with "certain diseases of early infancy." As a result, no comparison can be made with African Americans and white Americans. However, data is available for the general population of the United States, and although the comparison is between a small population (with relatively fewer deaths) and a large population, the comparison is revealing. In 1930, the death rate for the general population resulting from gastrointestinal disorders was 26, while it was 10 in 1940. In 1930 and 1940, Yakama death rates from gastrointestinal disorders were many times greater than that of the general population of the United States. As a cause of death, gastrointestinal disorders declined in the general population of the United States and on the Yakama Reservation. In 1950 and 1960, not one Yakama died of gastrointestinal disorders. However, they were an important cause of death among Yakama people during the first four decades of the twentieth century.[30]

Automobile Accidents

The best data available regarding automobile accidents, the sixth leading cause of death among Yakama people (N = 122/5.5 percent), are for the years 1920, 1940, and 1950, since no Yakama person was reported to have died as a result of automobile accidents in 1930 or 1960. The crude death rate per 100,000 resulting from automobile accidents in the Yakama population in 1920 was 34, while it was 5 among African Americans, 11 among white Americans, and 10 among the general population of the United States. In 1940, the Yakama had a crude death rate resulting from automobile accidents of 140, while the crude death rate was 24 among African Americans, 27 among white Americans, and 26 among the general population of the United States. In 1950, the Yakama suffered one fatality and had a crude death rate resulting from automobile accidents of 25 (figure 4.4). The larger perspective of Yakama deaths resulting from automobile accidents reveals that no Yakama person reportedly died while driving or riding in an automobile between 1888 and 1919. The first recorded Yakama fatality by automobile accident occurred in 1920 when a woman of 32 years of age was killed when a car hit her. It is not

known if she was in the car when she was hit. The first verifi-
able automobile fatality occurred in 1924 when a 45-year-old
male was riding in an automobile and was hit by another car.
He suffered a fractured skull and died from injuries.

Although 37 Yakama people died in automobile accidents
between 1924 and 1940, deaths by vehicular accidents did not
increase rapidly until after 1940. During the year of 1940, 5
people died in car accidents, and this was the sixth leading cause
of death on the reservation that year. The Yakama suffered
most often from automobile accidents after 1940, and particularly after 1946, in the post–World War II era, when Yakama
could afford to purchase and use more vehicles. One Yakama
died as a result of an automobile accident in 1950, but no
Yakama person died in an automobile accident in 1960,
although a total of 62 people died by this cause during the era
from 1950 to 1964 (figure 4.5). Of all deaths suffered by
Yakama people as a result of automobile accidents, 51 percent
took place from 1950 through 1964. Clearly, automobile accidents were a major cause of death among many different peoples of the United States during the twentieth century, including Yakama, but the number of Yakama deaths resulting from
automobile accidents rose sharply after 1950.[31]

Influenza

Influenza was the seventh leading cause of death among Yakama
Indians during the seventy-six year period (N = 104/5 percent).
In 1930 and 1960, no Yakama person was reported to have died
of influenza. However, a number of Yakama people died of
influenza in 1940, and a comparison for this year can be made
with the African American and white populations in the United
States. The death rate per 100,000 Yakama people who died of
influenza in 1940 was 84. The death rate among African Americans was 33, while it was 13 for whites (figure 4.4). Although
influenza killed individuals during other years covered by this
study, the best comparative data was found for 1940. Still,
influenza was not a frequent killer of Yakama in 1940 or any
year after 1933. It was, however, a major killer in 1918 as a
result of Spanish influenza, an epidemic that contributed to
deaths throughout the United States and the world.

In November 1918, Yakama Agent Donald M. Carr reported, "There is such an epidemic of grippe conditions among school children that the public schools in the County were closed the first weeks of October." He remarked that since 10 October 1918, "the disease spread with considerable rapidity."[32] Between 11 and 31 October 1918, Carr stated that 15 Yakama died. The Death Certificates indicate that a total of 17 Yakama died of influenza in 1918, which was 32 percent of all deaths in that year. Influenza was the foremost cause of death in 1918, and this was the most significant year in terms of deaths caused by influenza. It was a major killer only for the years before 1932. After that year, the number of Yakama deaths due to influenza dropped remarkably. However, influenza may have been a contributing factor for those Yakama who died of pneumonia and tuberculosis after 1932. Between 1933 and 1964, only 3 Yakama died of influenza. Death resulting from influenza was confined to the first three decades of the twentieth century, and this is probably due to the fact that the people received little health care until the 1920s when the national reform movement in Indian affairs affected the operation of the health division of the Office of Indian Affairs.[33]

Cancer

The eighth leading cause of death on the Yakama Reservation, cancer, was much less important as a cause of death among the Yakama people when compared to other populations of the United States (N = 82/3 percent). The low number of deaths resulting from cancer among Yakama is in marked contrast to the many deaths suffered by individuals in the general population of the United States, the African American population, and the white population. Most likely, diet and the use of tobacco had a great deal to do with the lower total number of deaths due to cancer.[34] While cancer was a leading cause of death among other populations in the United States after 1940, it was not a major cause of death on the Yakama Reservation during these years. In 1940, 2 Yakama died of cancer, and in 1950, 3 people died of it. In 1960, 1 person died of the disease. In the general population of the United States, cancer was the eighth leading cause of death in 1900 and the second major cause of death after 1940. As in the case of heart disease, there were fewer deaths by cancer among Yakama Indians than among other populations in the United States in the early part of the twentieth century, most likely because their diets during the first half of the twentieth century were lower in fats and the Indians used tobacco primarily for ceremonial purposes.

Among African Americans, cancer was the sixth leading cause of death in 1910, the third major cause of death in 1940, and the second most frequent cause of death in 1950 and 1960. Among white Americans, cancer was the fourth most frequent cause of death in 1910 and the second leading cause of death in both 1940 and 1960. Lung cancer was not a major cause of death among Yakama people, as Yakama suffered only 5 deaths due to lung cancer during the seventy-six year period from 1888 to 1964 (figure 4.4). Of the 82 Yakama people who died of cancer between 1925, when officials recorded the first death resulting from cancer, and 1964, 58 (71 percent) were women and 24 (29 percent) were men (figure 4.6). Of the 58 women who died of cancer, the principal types of cancer that caused deaths were cancer of the uterus (29 percent), stomach (24 percent), breast (16 percent), and cervix (5 percent). Thus, 34 percent of all cancer deaths suffered by women were reproductive system cancers, likely caused by infections induced by males who had multiple sex partners. However, doctors could not distinguish between cervical and uterine cancers without autopsies. These four types of cancer among females caused 74 percent of all cancer deaths experienced by Yakama women. Yakama men died of three major types of cancer, each causing 17 percent of male deaths. The cancers experienced most often by males included stomach, prostate-rectal, and general cancer. Clearly, Yakama women died more often than men of cancer, but neither suffered greatly from lung cancer.[35]

Premature Births

Premature births, a type of fetal death, ranked ninth as a cause of death on the Yakama Reservation (N = 64/3 percent). The number of deaths due to premature births is fairly evenly distributed from the 1920s to the 1960s. In spite of advances in medicine and the arrival of the Public Health Service on the reservation in the 1950s, the Yakama continued to suffer deaths caused by prematurity from 1950 through 1964 (N = 16/25 percent). It was important as a cause of death because premature births occurred so often within the Yakama population. The large number of deaths caused by prematurity contrasts with those found historically among the country's general population, African Americans, and white Americans in the United States. In 1940, 4 Yakamas died as a result of premature birth; in 1950, none; and in 1960, 2 fetuses died for this reason. Premature births were a leading cause of death during the years of the study, and "death by premature birth" was one of the ten leading causes of death on the Yakama Reservation between 1888 and 1964.

Premature births appear as the tenth leading cause of death within the general population of the United States for 1940, but it was not among the ten leading causes of death by 1960. Among African Americans, deaths resulting from premature births did not appear as one of the ten most important causes of death in the black population for 1910, 1940, or 1960. Among white Americans, premature birth was not among the ten most frequent causes of death for 1910, 1940, or 1960. In contrast, Yakama Indians suffered numerous deaths from premature births (Figure 3.10), although most of these occurred between the era from 1926 through 1937 (N = 22/34 percent). This was the period when Yakama and other Indians began experiencing the results of better public and medical health care resulting from the reform movements and advancements in medicine, but changes in health care were not reflected in the number of fetal deaths in the 1930s caused by premature births. Thus, among Yakama people, premature births continued as a serious cause of death.[36]

Senility and Old Age

The tenth most frequent cause of death on the Yakama Reservation was senility and old age (N = 57/3 percent). Senility was a cause of death used to denote the death of older Yakama men and women when family members, coroners, health officials, and doctors had no specific—clinical or medical—cause of death to record. In 1940, no Yakama died of senility or old age, and in 1960, only 1 person died from this cause. Nearly all Yakama that died of senility did so between 1925 and 1932. After 1932, this cause of death is listed only twice. This is likely due to advances in recording clinical causes of death on Death Certificates and medically determining more precisely the person's cause of death. Recorders of death used senility and old age as a cause of death because it was convenient when no other apparent cause of death was discovered for an elderly person. This cause of death does not appear as often as a leading cause of death among other populations within the United States.

Among the general population of the United States, senility ranked ninth as the leading cause of death in 1900, but it was not a major cause of death after 1940. Likewise, among the African American and white populations of the United States, senility does not appear as one of the ten leading causes of death for 1910, 1940, 1950, or 1960. The reason senility does not appear as a major cause of death in the other populations under review may well be the result of medical doctors' and coroners' carefully assessing causes of death, particularly deaths of elders, to determine the most likely cause of their deaths. The use of senility as a cause of death was a general designation for the death of older individuals, and it was easily applied in the early twentieth century to elders on the Yakama Reservation.

Analysis

An analysis of the leading causes of death on the Yakama Reservation for each ten–year interval reveals that tuberculosis was the major cause of death for each year included in the study until the 1940s when the number of deaths caused by tuberculosis dropped dramatically (figure 4.4). Deaths by tuberculosis declined significantly for the years between 1950 and 1964 because of preventive measures, public health, higher incomes, sanitation, housing improvements, medicines, and better health care for Indians. Of the 619 deaths from tuberculosis suffered by the Yakama between 1888 and 1964, 13 (2 percent) died between 1950 and 1964. This was a notable decrease in the number of deaths caused by tuberculosis compared to the years prior to 1950. However, pneumonia, the second leading cause of death for the seventy-six year period, did not decline as rapidly. Between 1950 and 1964, large numbers of Yakama people continued to die of pneumonia. Of the 566 people who died of pneumonia from 1888 to 1964, 125 (22 percent) died during the period from 1950 to 1964. Clearly, deaths caused by pneumonia in the 1950s and early 1960s far surpassed those caused by tuberculosis. Thus, pneumonia continued to be a conspicuous killer of Yakama people throughout much of the twentieth century.

While the number of deaths caused by tuberculosis declined in the 1940s and 1950s, deaths resulting from heart disease rose. Of the 325 people who died of heart diseases between 1888 and 1964, 127 (39 percent) of them did so between 1950 and 1964. Deaths by automobile accidents also rose after 1940 and were another important cause of death that emerged during the last fourteen years covered by this study. Between 1950 and 1964, the number of Yakama people that died in automobile accidents increased significantly. Of the 122 people who died as a result of automobile accidents, 62 (51 percent) did so between 1950 and 1964. During these same fourteen years of this study, heart disease became the foremost cause of death on the Yakama Reservation. In addition, cancer continued to be a primary cause of death on the reservation from 1950 to 1964, with 33 people dying of the disease. Of the Yakama who died of various cancers during the seventy-six year period, 40 percent did so during the last fourteen years of the era under examination. Thus heart disease, pneumonia, automobile accidents, and cancer were the major causes of death on the Yakama Reservation during the 1950s and early 1960s.

Causes of Death among Fetuses, Infants, and Children

Among the prevailing factors leading to the death of fetuses, infants, and children on the Yakama Indian Reservation were poor public health, lack of sanitation, and poverty. Scholars know a great deal about the traditional way of life of the Yakama prior to white contact, but death rates, fetal mortality rates, infant mortality rates, and other statistical information among the Yakama prior to white arrival in the Pacific Northwest are unknown. Generally, the Yakama lived comfortably, taking their livelihood from gathering, fishing, and hunting. After the introduction of horses (ca. 1750) and cattle (ca. 1830), the Yakama also lived by trading animals and ranching. The introduction of the reservation system by the United States radically changed the epidemiology and nutrition of Yakama people. It is more than likely that the reservation system, white settlement, changes in housing, settlement patterns of Euro-Americans, the lack of public health, and Indian policies designed to break traditional Indian patterns of life, so altered Yakama life that numerous native people died on the reservation. These changes occurred during the Age of Pestilence when numbers of Northwestern Indians died of contagious diseases brought by Euro-Americans.[37] The results of this transitional era were, in part, reflected in high fetal and infant mortality rates.[38]

It is reasonable to suggest from the data presented in this study that, diseases ravaged the Yakama population in the nineteenth and twentieth centuries and that the overall quality of life for the Yakama declined dramatically as a result of the reservation system. Native Americans, particularly infants, born on the reservation died in large numbers as a result of conditions on the reservation. However, there is no way to determine if native peoples living on the reservation suffered greater crude death rates or infant mortality rates than Indians living off the reservation. Before the reservation system, Indians lacked natural biological immunities to many diseases, and they died from many viral and bacterial diseases. The Yakama had little "medicine" with which to combat diseases brought by whites. The reservation system did not help the situation by providing new medicines and advanced health care. Instead, the reservation system created an unhealthy environment for Yakama people due to poor public health, absence of sanitation, harsh economic conditions, poor education, insufficient foods, inadequate health care, and social depression. Yakama people continued to be at risk in terms of death on the reservation during the first half of the twentieth century, and this was particularly true of fetuses and infants.

Fetal Deaths

Fetal deaths were common within the Yakama population during the first half of the twentieth century. Among Yakama people from 1888 to 1964, premature births (N = 64/61 percent) and stillbirths (N = 41/39 percent) were the key types of fetal deaths (figure 3.10). Premature births can be caused in many ways, and they occur when the birth of a baby takes place before 37 weeks' gestation.[39] The common term for premature births is miscarriages which occur when there is a separation of the fetus and placenta from the uterus. The cause of most miscarriages is simply not known, and the Death Certificates dealing with the Yakama are not detailed in this regard. Generally, state and county officials recording deaths on the Yakama Reservation stated that children died "prematurely."[40] A premature birth is generally more apt to occur if a mother has underlying medical problems, including diabetes, toxemia, or multiple fetuses.[41] Premature births can be caused by the early rupture of membranes surrounding the baby, and while this is a normal occurrence in full-term pregnancies, it is dangerous to the baby and mother, due to infection, if the membrane ruptures prematurely. Premature birth results, and this was the leading cause of fetal deaths among Yakama people.[42]

The Death Certificates indicate that stillbirth was the second leading explanation given for fetal deaths (N = 41). As stated above, stillbirth is an intrauterine death of a fetus when the baby is born dead after the twenty-eighth week of pregnancy.[43] Mothers with diabetes mellitus as well as those with toxemia may have a stillbirth. Stillbirth can also be caused by a hemorrhage or an abnormality in the fetus.[44] On the Yakama Reservation during the era from 1888 to 1964, premature birth and stillbirth accounted for the death of a total of 107 fetuses. Descriptions of death found in the Yakama Death Certificates caused by stillbirth vary. Most documents simply state "stillborn," but others state "died at birth," "Born Dead," "Slow Delivery of Head-Podal," "Stillbirth-Twisted Cord," or "Stillbirth—Breech Delivery."[45] Fetal deaths declined during the 1950s, in part because of prenatal medical education and advances in public health. Fewer fetal deaths occur in populations where prenatal care and preventive health education is provided, but Yakama received little health education or prenatal care until the 1950s. Preventive health care and education also influenced infant mortality rates and the well-being of infants under one year of age and children under six.

Infant and Children's Deaths

Between 1925 and 1964, pneumonia (figure 4.8) was the most dangerous disease among Yakama infants and children under six years of age (N = 347: males 215, females 132). They died of viral and bacterial pneumonia, although the distinction between the two types is not always given in the documents. Sometimes pneumonia was brought on by influenza viruses, but most often bacteria caused pneumonia. Pneumonia is an inflammation of the lungs, but other organs and parts of the body can become inflamed. In addition, children with pneumonia run high fevers, alternately experiencing chills and sweats. The disease is characterized by chest pains, coughing, and difficulty in breathing. Death results more often if children have an underlying condition such as malnutrition, infection, tuberculosis, or heart disease—all of which thrived on the Yakama Reservation. In these cases, pneumonia was the primary cause of death but other problems contributed to the body's weakened resistance which made the child susceptible to pneumonia. For Yakama children lacking natural immunities, pneumonia was deadly (figures 3.6, 3.7, 3.8).[46]

Like pneumonia, gastrointestinal disorders were important causes of death among infants and children under six years of age (N = 108: males 65, females 43). In Yakama children, disorders of the digestive tract proved fatal, particularly if infections were present. The fundamental reason pneumonia and gastrointestinal diseases developed within the infant population of the Yakama was that bacilli and viruses flourished in the reservation environment where public health and sanitation were poor or nonexistent throughout much of the early twentieth century. Antibiotics were scarce on the reservation or simply not available until the 1930s, and children without medicines to fight bacterial infections often died. The stomach, intestines, and other parts of the digestive tract naturally contain essential bacteria for life, but sometimes dangerous bacilli invade the body, multiply rapidly, and infect the gut wall then entering the bloodstream and spreading to other parts of the body. Gastrointestinal infections were nearly always caused by bacteria, and children infected with such disorders suffered one or more symptoms, including abdominal and intestinal pain, cramps, diarrhea, fever, and vomiting. Most often children become dehydrated, and although they are thirsty, they are unable to keep the fluids in their stomachs.[47]

Another common killer of Yakama children was tuberculosis (N = 66: females 39, males 27).[48] Although the disease normally takes time to develop, it could grow rapidly in some hosts and kill the person, particularly infants suffering from malnutrition or other disease. Tuberculosis was one of the most prominent causes of death among Yakama children, but it preyed far more on young adults between 15 and 29 years of age. Tuberculosis is caused by airborne bacilli which generally spread from one person to another, landing in the lungs where the bacilli multiply and destroy tissues.[49] Tubercule bacilli are usually attacked by natural antibodies, and if they are not destroyed, they can spread to other body parts. Bacilli may react to antibodies, but if children are malnourished or have a low resistance, the tubercle bacilli can travel to other parts of the body through the blood and lymph nodes, attacking other organs.[50] For months or years tubercle bacilli can travel about the body but remain dormant. This process can linger for some time as bacilli remain inactive, but bacilli can also become active at any point. In small children, tubercle bacilli can take hold quickly, particularly if children are ill, undernourished, or living in unsanitary or overcrowded housing.

In a recent study of lung and lymph tissue taken from the body of a Peruvian Indian woman believed to have lived 1,000 years ago, scholars of the University of Minnesota determined from genetic studies "that tuberculosis was not introduced into the Americas by Europeans." This was a theory long held by some scholars, but the physical evidence of the tissue is revealing and appears definitive. Tuberculosis existed in the Americas prior to 1492, but there is no evidence that it existed among the Yakama prior to white contact. However, if tuberculosis did exist among the Yakama, it is not believed to have developed into epidemic proportions among the Yakama until after the 1860s when the United States forced fourteen distinct tribes and bands onto the Yakama Reservation. Wilmar L. Salo, a scholar working for the University of Minnesota, pointed out that "the harsh treatment of the Indians doubtless contributed to the American epidemic of the disease."[51] And he is correct. By changing the way Indians lived, Europeans, and later, officials of the United States, created a climate that encouraged the spread of tuberculosis.

According to Selman Waksman, American Indians suffered severely because they were "confined to barracks or permanent reservation quarters" where they showed "a marked rise in tuberculosis rate which far exceed that of either Negro or white persons." He also argued that the semi-nomadic life of many Native Americans was conducive to good health, free from the ravages of tuberculosis. Children and young adults were particularly affected by the disease, and when they suffered with tuberculosis, they experienced fatigue, fever, and loss of appetite. They usually had a dry cough producing phlegm filled with blood and pus. Tuberculosis also spread as a result of contact with sputum, pus, and blood. Patients coughed and spit, spreading the bacilli onto others, into the air, bed clothing, blankets, and other material items. Dishes, eating utensils, and cups became contaminated, and the disease spread uncontrollably from patient to family to friends. Children carried tuberculosis to school, social events, powwows, and church, innocently spreading it among the larger reservation population. When tuberculosis strikes, children lose weight, and they can develop lumps in their bodies from swollen lymph nodes. Many Yakama children had secondary causes of death, including tuberculosis, but often the primary cause of their demise was tuberculosis, a disease that ravaged Native American populations during the first half of the twentieth century because of poor living conditions, malnutrition, and a host of other infectious diseases that preyed on native peoples, making them more susceptible to tuberculosis.[52]

Miscellaneous accidents were another cause of death among Yakama children (N = 17: males 10, females 7).[53] Examples of accidental deaths include "accident—after taking ether anesthetic for operation," "drowned in irrigation ditch," and "injuries, multiple, extreme, Impact of train." Others included "accidental gunshot wound," "rattlesnake bite," and "Asphyxia, Drowning; Fell in creek while playing."[54] Not surprisingly, accidental deaths occurred most often for children one year to six because of their increased mobility. It does not appear as a major cause of death among infants under one year of age.

Syphilis also contributed to the death of children on the Yakama Reservation, and it was primarily a cause of death among infants (N = 12: male infants 9, female infants 3). Syphilis is a sexually transmitted disease caused by a bacterium known as *treponema pallidum*. On the Yakama Reservation, syphilis was transmitted between adult sexual partners and from mothers to their fetuses. When the disease went untreated, syphilis killed Yakama infants. Among the Yakama, the disease appeared in that age group of children under one year of age, and syphilis was the fifth leading cause of death among Yakama infants. In addition to the 12 infants who died of the disease, 2 other children (2 males, one and two years old) under six years of age died of syphilis. Also, 2 females twenty–four years of age and 2 males in their 60s died of syphilis.

Whooping cough was another cause of death among children (N = 7: males 4, females 3). It was most important as a cause of death among Yakama in that age category of children one year of age. The disease is caused by a bacillus that infects the lungs, clogging air passages with thick mucus. Symptoms develop between seven and fourteen days after children are infected, appearing like an ordinary cold with coughing and fever but continuing without abatement. Nasal discharges become thick, and coughing increases. Children with whooping cough have trouble breathing, because oxygen is restricted from moving freely in and out of the lungs. Sometimes children vomit after coughing spells. They also gasp for air after severe coughing, making a whooping noise from which the disease derives its name. Living in poverty and without immunization, public health programs or sanitation, Yakama children were susceptible to whooping cough, and some of them died of the disease.[55]

Other Yakama children, especially those in the age group under six but older than two, died of meningitis, a contagious disease. Meningitis affects the three thin layers that cover the brain and are known as the meninges. Children with meningitis suffer from an infection which they contract from another person.[56] Sometimes the disease is linked to tuberculosis and mumps, although it generally occurs alone. When children are infected with the disease, they develop headaches. They will arch their sore necks backward and seem irritable, refusing to move their heads forward because of severe pain. In infants, the front of the head bulges and the child may vomit. Because meningitis is usually a bacterial infection, antibiotics can treat the disease.[57] Although, Alexander Fleming discovered penicillin in 1928, antibiotics were not available to fight bacilli that caused many contagious diseases, including meningitis, until the 1930s, and even then, antibiotics and preventive serums were often scarce on the Yakama Reservation. Medical attention was also difficult to obtain due to the lack of doctors, nurses, and hospitals. Moreover, public health programs did not develop fully on the reservation until the Indian New Deal era of the 1930s and early 1940s. Yakama children died as a result.

In addition to the major causes of death among Yakama children under six years of age, there were several minor causes of death worthy of note. The most notable of these minor causes of death were automobile accidents, heart disease, suffocation, and measles.[58] Children who died in automobile accidents were generally inside the car, traveling as passengers, but a few of them were hit by automobiles. All of the automobile-related deaths were coded in this category. Suffocation may have provided a way for recorders to note deaths resulting from sudden infant death syndrome or "crib death."[59] When an infant died suddenly, and there was no other apparent cause, officials recorded the cause of death as "suffocation," a designation most prominent in the age category from birth to one year of age. Infant death syndrome has been a significant cause of death among Native American infants during the 1980s and 1990s.

Heart disease and measles were also minor causes of death among children under six years of age, and they appeared sufficiently often to warrant note. Heart disease includes many disorders such as diseases of the valves, congenital heart disease, heart attacks, heart failure, and others. Most childhood deaths involving the heart were congenital heart disease or abnormality of the heart at the time of birth. Congenital heart disease can be caused in the fetus if the mother has an infection or contracts German measles (rubella) while she is pregnant. Some disorders of the heart are genetic, including Down's syndrome and Marfan's syndrome, the latter of which is a disorder of the collagen or protein fibrous tissue that strengthens the vessels, valves, and heart. Although these syndromes likely developed

among children on the Yakama Reservation, none of the Death
Certificates specifically identify them as a cause of death. Instead, the documents list heart disease, heart failure, or congenital heart disease as causes of heart-related deaths among
children.[60]

Measles appeared as a notable cause of death only for children one year of age. Once a common killer among American
Indians, measles declined in importance during the second half
of the nineteenth century. In 1847, the disease triggered a major
uprising of Cayuse Indians against Marcus and Narcissa Whitman, missionaries to the Cayuse at Waiilatpu—the Place of the
Rye Grass. In 1848, following the dangerous measles epidemic,
war broke out between the Cayuse and Palouse Indians and
Oregon Volunteers. Although the Yakama did not participate
in the Whitman killings or the war, they were aware of the
problems associated with the dreaded disease known to whites
as measles.[61] However, by the twentieth century, measles (like
smallpox) was not an important cause of death among the
Yakama people. It was not among the top five diseases that
took the lives of Yakama children in any age category from
1888 to 1964, although it ranked eighth as a cause of death
among Yakama children one year of age.

Overview

During the early twentieth century, Yakama people lived
through the last stages of the Age of Pestilence, although they
were no longer significantly plagued by smallpox, measles, and
fevers. Instead, the last stages of the Age of Pestilence and the
Age of Receding Pandemics saw Yakama children suffering
from pneumonia, gastrointestinal disorders, tuberculosis, syphilis, whooping cough, and meningitis (figures 3.6, 3.7, 3.8, 4.8).[62]
Also, throughout the twentieth century, children faced several
deaths through miscellaneous and automobile accidents. Most
of these causes were influenced by factors surrounding life on
the reservation where poverty flourished. Poor diets, lack of
public health, little medical care, unsanitary housing, and social
anomie contributed to all of the leading causes of death suffered
by Yakama fetuses, infants, and children.[63] Moreover, the
health division of the Office of Indian Affairs did not

adequately educate native people about the cause and prevention of disease or provide them with sufficient prenatal care so that infants would be born healthy, prepared to face life-threatening diseases and challenges that thrived on the Yakama Reservation.

Fetuses, infants, and children on the reservation were also at risk because of the lack of medicine, doctors, nurses, and hospitals. They were at risk because mothers received little or no prenatal care or basic education about sanitation, disease prevention, disease control, and techniques of quarantining infants, children, and other patients. They were at risk because parents no longer ate as many traditional foods or served them to their children. The Yakama Reservation became a host for bacilli and viruses that wreaked havoc on infants and children who were undernourished and who lived in cramped, unsanitary homes. Bacteria especially spread rapidly through the air and on such material items as blankets, bedding, cups, flatware, dishes, and clothing. They thrived in homes where people were unaccustomed to cleaning themselves, their houses, and material items with soap, water, and disinfectants, since they had never needed to do so before the introduction of so many new and deadly bacteria. They did not understand germ theory, and as a result, bacilli spread quickly from person to person, spreading pneumonia, tuberculosis, and a variety of gastrointestinal disorders. In addition to disease, the reservation system also created circumstances that contributed to accidental deaths among small children.

Fetuses, infants, and children were also at risk because of nutritional changes among adults and children alike, particularly expectant mothers whose health greatly influenced their offspring at every stage of development. When the government of the United States forced fourteen diverse tribes and bands onto the reservation, the government broke a pattern of life that had been established at the time of Yakama creation, when humans formed a spiritual, physical, and cultural relationship with salmon, deer, roots, berries, and other foods. In the early twentieth century, the government ended seasonal rounds of Indians, compelling them more and more to remain on the reservation rather than moving from root to fishing to hunting grounds on and off the reservation. The government broke the natural cycle of the people which had profound health implications. In addition to detrimental changes in diet, the government altered familial and band relationships. As Indians became more sedentary, grandmothers, mothers, aunts, and other relatives who once shared in the caring of children no longer banded together as regularly to travel from the rivers to plateaus and from plateaus to mountains.

The ties between women who cared for each other's children through extended families and extended relationships were changed by the reservation system which encouraged or required Indians to remain in certain areas where extended family and friends may or may not have been located. Furthermore, the reservation altered the role of women who had once gathered a preponderant amount of natural fruits and vegetables. Although women continued to gather some roots and berries, they generally ran their family's affairs on the reservation through ranching, farming, and wage earning. Women gradually did not share as many child-care duties and had to work outside of the home for the survival of the family. One of the consequences of this was the accidental death of children after they had reached one year of age. Working mothers could not provide for their families and watch their children, and without a familial support system among the women to care for children, the children put themselves in harm's way and some of them died as a result of accidents. Working mothers who no longer traveled in seasonal rounds with other women witnessed a change in prenatal care, birthing, and postnatal care. Prior to the reservation system, midwives and female assistants aided with pregnancies and deliveries, but agents discouraged old traditions, and forced settlement by Indians on the reservation diminished the interaction of women with midwives and other women trained in birthing. This was yet another circumstance associated with infant deaths on the reservation.

The reservation system of the United States destroyed the native standard of living and introduced a host of viruses and bacilli to the Indians living on the Yakama Reservation. The result was poverty, ill health, and death among Yakama people. Once the United States had destroyed much of Indian culture, they failed to enrich it in accordance with trust and treaty responsibilities by providing minimal health care for native people living on the Yakama Reservation. Without housing, public health, sanitation, education, medicine, doctors, nurses, sanitoriums, and hospitals, and living in a state of social disarray, and depression, Yakama women were vulnerable to premature births and stillbirths. Yakama infants and children fell victim to pneumonia, tuberculosis, gastrointestinal disorders, accidental deaths, and a variety of diseases that also took the lives of many fetuses.

Fetal and Infant Deaths

During much of the twentieth century, Yakama people suffered from high fetal and infant mortality. According to John Weeks, fetuses and infants are "fragile and completely dependent on others for survival." Within the Yakama society, this fragility and dependency of unborn and newborn babies are reflected in the high incidences of mortality. Comparison of fetal and infant mortality among the Yakama, whites in the United States, non-whites in the United States, and the population of Washington state illuminates the fact that Yakama Indians lived in poverty. They had little or no formal education—depending on the era and the gender of the individual—and they had little income. In spite of the Yakama treaty, Yakama people lived in poverty and endured a multitude of social, economic, educational, and health problems that contributed to a higher number of deaths than that experienced by other populations[64]

It is clear from the Yakama Death Certificates for the years 1888 through 1964 that the most deadly age within the population of Yakama Indians was under during the first twelve months after being born (figure 3.9). The first year of life is a dangerous time among many world populations, particularly among people living under the conditions described. Examination of the Death Certificates indicates that between 1888 and 1964, the Yakama experienced a total of 737 (19 percent) fetal and infant deaths. This is the largest number of deaths recorded in any age group.

Fetal Deaths

Officials recorded two types of fetal deaths in the Death Certificates: premature births and stillbirths (figure 3.10). Those children that died before birth have been separated from infants and constitute fetal deaths. Thus, causes of death for fetuses are not included in the five leading causes of death among children under one year of age, because these babies were not born alive. Of these children, 64 died of premature birth and 43 were stillborn. Among the Yakama, more males than females were born prematurely or were stillborn, a development common in many populations, since females are hardier biologically than males. Of those fetuses that died of premature birth, 38 (60 percent) were males and 26 (40 percent) were females. Most of these deaths are related to causes associated with poverty. However, some of them are linked to the general conditions of the Yakama Nation in the early twentieth century which was one of social depression or anomie. The population suffered from many diseases and deaths, and individuals living on the reservation had little hope for the future. These native people had been militarily defeated in the middle of the nineteenth century, and they had lived under the yoke of white bureaucrats during the late nineteenth and early twentieth centuries. Their lives were inextricably tied to the United States, and so they suffered during the 1920s and 1930s from the Depression. Parents and grandparents watched the Indian Office force their children into government schools off the reservations—schools designed to destroy Indian languages and cultures. The general health of Yakama people, including pregnant mothers or those dealing with newborns, was tied to the state of affairs within the Yakama world and that of the larger white population.[65]

High rates of fetal deaths on the Yakama Reservation were of concern to officials of the Office of Indian Affairs. With limited funding, the Office of Indian Affairs instructed Indian agents to use portions of their budgets to combat fetal and infant deaths, but the funding to educate mothers about pre- and postnatal care was not sufficient or continual.[66] An examination of the "Health & Hospitalization Records and Reports, 1912–1940" in the National Archives, Pacific Northwest Region, demonstrates that the Yakama Agency sponsored a few health workshops in the early twentieth century. The lack of additional workshops and preventive care programs was due to the absence of funds from Washington, D. C., and insufficient staff. From letters written in the agency letterbooks, it appears that some agents were genuinely concerned about the problem of fetal and infant deaths on the Yakama Reservation. In 1917, for example, Yakama Agent Donald M. Carr supported the efforts of Field Matron Esther M. Sprague to meet and discuss with Yakama mothers "caring and proper feeding of children and cleanliness." This was all part of a "Baby Week" program on the reservation in 1917, and it educated mothers about caring for themselves and their babies.[67] Agent Carr and Field Matron Sprague offered their program to 26 Yakama women in 1917, but funds were not available for a full-scale, on-going project to provide pre- and postnatal education for women on the reservation.[68]

Yakama mothers lacked prenatal care and education which was supposed to be provided by the medical component of the Office of Indian Affairs. With the reservation system came a change in the Yakama way of life that prevented women from interacting with other women as they moved across the Columbia Plateau to hunt, gather, and fish. Mothers who had once moved in bands across the Columbia Plateau in pursuit of roots, berries, fish, and game, no longer came into contact as often with medicine men and women. No longer could mothers easily turn to experienced midwives and elders trained in the use of medicinal plants for advice, medicine, and treatment. Also, confinement on the reservation limited the amount of traditional foods mothers ate, including nutritious fruits and vegetables that were high in vitamins. In general, the common and traditional skills of medicine people and midwives declined with the "new white order" brought to Yakama lands by agents of the Indian Office. Thus, to some degree, traditional foods and medicines gave way, as the government forced Indians into new modes of life. Nutrition declined and so did the amount of available food and variety of food sources. These changes led to medical problems and the deterioration of the general health of mothers and their unborn children. Without foods, public health, sanitation, and medical attention, the health of pregnant women declined, and the harvest was premature births and stillborn babies.[69]

Fetal Mortality Rate

An analysis of fetal death rates per 1,000 live births in the population indicates that the Yakama generally had higher fetal death rates than whites in the United States from 1926 to 1946 (figures 3.5, 4.9). During this twenty-year period, Yakama had a peak fetal death rate per 1,000 live births in 1926 with a rate of 194, in comparison to whites who had a rate of 35. The fetal death rate among Yakama declined slightly to 70 per 1,000 live births in 1928, perhaps in response to the national Indian reform movement and the publication of the *Meriam Report*. In 1929, the Yakama fetal death rate dropped remarkably to 27 which was less than the death rate of 34 experienced by whites in the United States. However, after 1929, the Yakama fetal death rate climbed again to 36 in 1930, 60 in 1931, and 143 in 1936. A moving average of fetal death rates among Yakama and whites in the United States reveals that from 1926 through 1949, the Yakama experienced a fetal death rate many times greater than whites in the United States, but between 1950 and 1959, the Yakama had a fetal death rate below whites. This was likely due to greater attention to public health and better medical health care offered by the Public Health Service in the 1950s. However, Yakama fetal death rate per 1,000 live births rose between 1960 and 1964 to a level above that of whites but not above non-whites in the United States.

A comparison of fetal death rates among the Yakama and non-whites in the United States is illuminating. This category of "non-whites" was created and used by the United States Census Bureau, and it is used here in discussing statistical data associated with African Americans, Latinos, Native Americans, Asian Americans, and other minority people deemed "non-white" by the Census Bureau. A comparison of the Yakama and non-white population of the United States reveals an erratic pattern in which the Yakama had a higher fetal death rate per 1,000 live births in selected years, and non-whites had a higher fetal death rate in other years. The former is the case from 1926 to 1943. However, after 1944, non-whites had a pattern of fetal death rates higher than that of Yakama people. This was probably the result of national reforms in American Indian health and general policies brought about by the Indian New Deal of the 1930s and early 1940s. Averages of fetal death rates were calculated by adding the rates for each year at five-year intervals, and this was done to smooth out the statistical data that was often erratic due to the fact that the Yakama population was small. The moving averages from 1920 to 1964 reveal much the same pattern as the fetal death rate, with a major change occurring after the era from 1945 to 1949, when non-whites consistently had a higher fetal death rate than Yakama people.

Clearly, before the 1940s, the fetal death rate among the Yakama was most often higher than among whites and frequently higher than among non-whites in the United States. Between 1940 and 1964, the fetal death rate of the Yakama remained below that of non-whites in the United States. This change in fetal death rates among Yakama after the 1940s may reflect improvements in public and medical health care, diet, and housing, as well as a greater emphasis on prenatal care. It may also reflect an improvement in funding for health and medicine for Native Americans and on the Yakama Reservation during and after World War II. However, Hunn has questioned the decline in the overall number of deaths on the Yakama Reservation during the 1940s and 1950s, suggesting that it may also be due to a change in the recording of deaths. He may be correct. During the 1940s, the government was preoccupied with the Second World War and recovery after the war, not the accounting of Indian deaths. Furthermore, in the 1950s, the government was more interested in terminating its trust relationship with tribes or relocating Indians to urban areas than it was in keeping vital statistics on native people. Perhaps these national developments had something to do with the decrease in the number of fetal and infant deaths reported in Yakama Death Certificates.

Infant Deaths

Between 1888 and 1964, officials recorded that 737 deaths occurred within the Yakama Indian population under one year of age. This number includes 106 fetal deaths recorded in the Death Certificates, which means that the Yakama suffered 631 infant deaths during the seventy-six-year period. Of these infants, 327 (52 percent) died of five leading causes. The foremost killer of Yakama infants was pneumonia which took the lives of 215 (34 percent) children under one year of age (figure 3.6). Of these deaths by pneumonia, 141 (66 percent) were males, while 74 (34 percent) were females (figure 4.10). The disease was sometimes brought on by influenza or a viral infection of the lungs. Infants living in an environment without public health, in substandard and unsanitary housing, and with inadequate health care fell victim to pneumonia and died in large numbers.[70] Pneumonia was the leading cause of death among Yakama Indian infants, and males had a significantly larger number of deaths by this cause than did females. Within the entire Yakama population during the seventy-six-year period, children within the category under four years of age recorded 344 of the total of 566 deaths by pneumonia. Thus, Yakama children under five years of age suffered 61 percent of all deaths caused by pneumonia within the Yakama population.

Gastrointestinal disorders caused the death of 66 (10 percent) infants during the era under examination (figure 3.6). This was the second leading cause of death among children under one year of age. Gastrointestinal disorders took the lives of 37 (56 percent) females and 29 (44 percent) males. Within the general Yakama population from 1888 to 1964, children in that category from 0-4 years of age experienced 105 of the 124 deaths resulting from gastrointestinal disorders. Therefore, 85 percent of all deaths suffered by the Yakama as a result of gastrointestinal disorders were those deaths among children under five years of age. Yakama infants and children under five years of age died often of gastrointestinal disorders including gastroenteritis, vomiting, diarrhea, and infections of the stomach, intestines, and other areas of the digestive tract. Yakama children died of dehydration and diarrhea, two major elements of gastrointestinal disorders which took the lives of many children from diverse populations around the world. Among Yakama infants, gastrointestinal disorders were the second leading cause of death. Tuberculosis was the third.

Between 1888 and 1964, a total of 18 (3 percent) infants died of tuberculosis (figure 3.6). Officials recording these deaths on the Death Certificates most often indicated that the infant had died of "tuberculosis," rarely specifying which type of tuberculosis. Occasionally, the certificates noted that the infant had died of "pulmonary tuberculosis," even though the disease could attack an infant's brains, lungs, kidneys, bones, or other parts of the body. However, it was difficult for family members, physicians, or coroners to know the extent of tuberculosis within the body without an autopsy, and autopsies were seldom, if ever, conducted. Of the 18 infants that died of tuberculosis, 10 (56 percent) were females and 8 (44 percent) were males. The fact that more female than male infants among the Yakama died of tuberculosis corresponded to a trend in the general population of the Yakama. On the Yakama Reservation during the seventy-six year period, females died of tuberculosis more often than males by a 54 to 46 percent margin, roughly the same margin as that reflected among Yakama children under one year of age. In their study entitled *The White Plague*, the Dubos point out that females have two times a greater rate of infection than males, although the reasons are unclear. However, the Yakama population was typical of this trend, since female infants, children, and adults died more often than males of tuberculosis.[71]

Infants and younger children did not suffer from tuberculosis as much as older children and young adults. During the seventy-six year period in question, children in the category under four years of age experienced 56 (9 percent) of all deaths caused by tuberculosis. In contrast, that group of 15-19 years of age had 112 (18 percent) of the deaths caused by tuberculosis. A total of 43 percent of all tuberculosis deaths occurred among Yakama people from ages between 15 and 29. Throughout the Yakama population, deaths resulting from tuberculosis were the result of exposure to tubercle bacilli, malnutrition, the lack of public health, unsanitary living conditions, and inadequate medical care. Although tuberculosis was a leading cause of death among Yakama children under one year of age, it was not as devastating to this age group as it was to older children and young adults.

Heart disease was the fourth major cause of death among Yakama infants, taking the lives of 16 (3 percent) children under one year of age. Of these infants, 9 (56 percent) were females and 6 (44 percent) were males, with 1 infant's gender unknown. In the case of tuberculosis, this was roughly the same percentage seen throughout the era under examination for the general population of the Yakama, with females leading males in the number of heart-related deaths by a margin of 52 to 48 percent. Most of the heart-related deaths that occurred within the Yakama population occurred among the very young and the old, namely Yakama over fifty-five years of age. Within the group under four years of age, 20 (6 percent) deaths occurred, and of this number, 16 were experienced by children under one year of age. Yakama children under five years of age had more heart–related deaths than any other age group from birth through 54 years of age. Heart diseases of all types were responsible for many deaths among infants under one year of age and children under four.

Finally, syphilis was the fifth leading cause of death among Yakama infants. All of the infants who died of the deadly disease contracted it while in utero. A total of 12 (2 percent) children under one year of age died of syphilis, and of this number, 9 (75 percent) were males and 3 (25 percent) were females. During the years from 1888 to 1964, a total of 19 Yakama people died of syphilis. Of this number, 12 were infants and 15 were children in the group under four years of age. Thus, 79 percent of all Yakama that died of syphilis were children who had contracted the disease from their mothers. During the same time period, only two adults died of the disease. While syphilis was among the five major causes of death among Yakama infants, it was only one of many varied causes of death that contributed to a high infant mortality rate among Yakama people. A total of 70 percent of all infant deaths among Yakama people occurred between 1924 and 1945, and the largest number of infant deaths in a single year occurred in 1931 when 36 children under one year of age died on the Yakama Reservation. Only 28 percent of the infant deaths on the reservation occurred between 1946 and 1964, and the number of infant deaths dropped dramatically after World War II as a result of antibiotics, improved health care, and economic improvements (figure 4.11).

Infant Mortality Rate

Birth records for native peoples living on the Yakama Indian Reservation were available for all the years between 1914 and 1964, except for the years 1915, 1916, 1917, 1920, 1922, 1924, and 1925. The first year for which death and birth records were available for analysis was 1914, but in this year, officials recorded only two live births and one death of an infant under one year of age. Better data exists for most years after 1914, and an infant mortality rate was calculated for every year that data was available. An infant mortality rate is the number of deaths of children under one year of age per 1,000 live births in the population, excluding premature births and stillbirths. Two interesting exceptions are in 1924 and 1925, for the birth and death documents indicate that the Yakama had more deaths of infants under one year of age than they had live births, which illustrates some of the recording problems found in the early data. In 1924, the records show 8 births and 14 deaths; in 1925, the documents show 6 births and 22 deaths. The data was drawn from two distinct sources, Birth Registers and Death Certificates, both of which are preserved in the National Archives, Pacific Northwest Region. In 1924 and 1925, either the Yakama did not report the births of their babies or officials collecting the data missed several births. For years in which sufficient data was available, an infant mortality rate was calculated and compared to whites and non-whites in the United States as well as the general population of Washington, the state surrounding the Yakama Nation.

The most complete data on births and deaths on the Yakama Indian Reservation was found for the years between 1926 and 1964. During this time period, the Yakama experienced their highest infant mortality rate in 1927, when they had a rate of 684 per 1,000 live births in the population. By comparison, that same year, whites in the United States had an infant mortality rate of 61, non-whites had a rate of 100, and the people of Washington had a rate of 50. Therefore, the Yakama had an infant mortality rate significantly higher than that of other populations within the United States (figure 4.12). This comparison is useful as a way of illustrating the high rate of infant mortality on the reservation within the boundaries of the United States and the state of Washington.

An examination of the infant mortality rates experienced by Yakama people and whites within the United States demonstrates that, with the exception of 1948 (a year in which officials may have failed to record the exact number of infant deaths), the Yakama had a higher infant mortality rate than whites over a period of forty years. This trend is also evident in the comparison between the infant mortality rate of the Yakama and that of the people of Washington. Again, except for the year 1948, the Yakama had an infant mortality rate higher than the people of Washington. Indeed, in most years, the infant mortality rate of the Yakama was many times higher.

Although the amount of difference is not as great, over a period of four decades, the Yakama experienced an infant mortality rate per 1,000 live births higher than that of non-whites in the United States. However, the infant mortality rate of the Yakama declined generally over the years from 1926 to 1964, dropping continually below 100 deaths per 1,000 live births after 1955. This was likely due to a general improvement of Yakama health in the 1940s and 1950s as well as better public and medical health care provided by the Public Health Service after 1954.

As was the case with fetal death rates, the infant mortality rates for the Yakama are erratic. Therefore, moving averages of infant mortality rates were calculated for the years in which data was available from 1920 to 1964. The data shows a general and steady decline in the infant mortality rate of Yakama from 1925 to 1964, except for a slight rise during the five-year period between 1940 and 1944. This rise in infant mortality rates may have been related to World War II, a time when Yakama men and women went off to war or worked in defense-related activities that may have placed fetuses and newborn babies at risk. Overall the moving averages depicting infant mortality rates on the Yakama Reservation declined from a high of 497 per 1,000 live births during the years from 1925 to 1929 to 52 per 1,000 live births during the years from 1960 to 1964. This is an important decline, and like the decline in fetal deaths, it may have been due to an improved standard of living on the reservation and better health care.

In their penetrating study of childhood mortality entitled *Fatal Years*, Preston and Haines argue that child mortality was higher in urban areas than rural areas.[72] They based their conclusion on census data in the United States for 1900, and although this assumption holds true for the population of the United States in 1900, it is not operative during the early twentieth century when dealing with Yakama (and possibly other reservation Indians), a population that resides in a rural setting. Unlike urban populations of the time, the Yakama population of 1900 was relatively untouched by the industrial revolution that characterized eastern urban centers, and yet the Yakama suffered high infant mortality throughout most of the early twentieth century. Preston and Haines point out that, in 1900, foreign-born children in urban areas had higher mortality than native born children, and Yakama infants mirrored foreign-born children and suffered higher infant mortality than non-native children born in the United States.[73] The moving average of infant mortality rates demonstrate the fact that the infant mortality rate within the Yakama Indian population was consistently higher than that of whites and non-whites within the United States as well as the people of the Washington state.

The moving averages of fetal and infant mortality rates show that the highest rates of death occurred from roughly the 1920s to 1945 (figures 4.11, 4.12,4.13). This was also the result of the Great Depression which struck rural areas in the 1920s before the stock market crash. The general health of Yakama people was poor during this era, a condition connected, in part, to the economic problems of the state and nation. The Yakama Nation was situated in an area heavily tied to ranching and agriculture, and since both of these economic pursuits suffered in the 1920s and 1930s, so did Yakama people. Lives of Yakama people were also tied to national reforms in Indian affairs during this same time period. The reformers did not push their agenda until the 1920s, and their efforts did not bear fruit until the late 1930s and early 1940s. However, their efforts had many tangible results, including a gradual improvement in economic, political, and public health, and in educational matters pertaining to Native Americans. A reflection of this is apparent in the improvement of health on the Yakama Reservation and the lowering of fetal and infant mortality rates after World War II.[74]

Another factor had a bearing on fetal and infant mortality rates on the Yakama Reservation. This was the passage in 1954 of Public Law 83–568, a bill known as the Transfer Act, which transferred the health care of American Indians and Alaskan Natives from the Bureau of Indian Affairs to the Department of Health, Education, and Welfare, known today as the Department of Health and Human Services. Throughout most of the twentieth century, the Public Health Service had aided the Interior Department in its efforts to deliver health care to Native Americans, but after 1954, the Public Health Service took full command of health delivery among Indian people.[75] Health care improved, and this is evident in lower fetal and infant mortality rates in comparison to most years before the 1950s. Still, over the course of much of the twentieth century, the Yakama witnessed numerous deaths of fetuses and infants. Although the comparison is between a small population and a large population, it is revealing that the average fetal mortality rate between 1926 and 1964 among the Yakama per 1,000 live births was 42, while, during the same period, it was 23 among whites in the United States. The infant mortality rate among the Yakama was even worse. During the course of forty-two years, the Yakama experienced an average infant mortality rate per 1,000 live births of 198, while, during the same years whites in the United States had an infant mortality rate of 41. Thus, the Yakama had a fetal mortality rate that was nearly double that of whites in the United States and suffered an infant mortality rate nearly five times greater than that of whites in the country.

Mortality among Yakama Children One Year of Age

Yakama children who were one year of age suffered the second largest number of deaths on the Yakama Reservation between 1888 and 1964. According to the Death Certificates, a total of 235 (6 percent) children died at the age of one. Of the children who died in this age category, 128 (54 percent) were males and 101 (43 percent) were females, with the gender of six children unknown.[76] As was the case for infants under one year of age, one-year-olds suffered most severely from pneumonia. This was the leading cause of death for children one year of age (figure 3.7). A total of 62 (44 percent) children died of pneumonia while one year of age. Pneumonia was a major killer of one year olds, but the number of children who died of the disease was dramatically lower than the 215 (41 percent) babies under one year of age who died from the same cause. However, the percentage of children of one year of age who died of pneumonia actually increased. Of those children one year old who died of pneumonia, 37 (60 percent) were males and 25 (40 percent) were females, which was a gender split approximately the same as it was for children under one year of age. In both cases, males died more often than females because of the biological superiority of female infants over male infants.

Among Yakama children of one year of age, gastrointestinal disorders followed pneumonia as the leading cause of death (figure 3.7). Gastrointestinal disorders took the lives of 27 (19 percent) children in this age category. As in the case with pneumonia, the number of children who died of gastrointestinal disorders was less than that reported for children under one year of age, but the percentage of death by gastrointestinal disorders also increased for those children one year of age. Of those children one year of age who died of gastrointestinal disorders, 16 (59 percent) were males and 11 (41 percent) were females. In terms of percentages, this is a similar gender split as that for infants under one year of age, with males dying more often than females. Stomach, intestinal, and digestive disorders were followed by tuberculosis as the third major cause of death among Yakama children one year of age.

A total of 15 (11 percent) children one year old died of tuberculosis, again a lower number of deaths than for infants under one year old (figure 3.7). However, a larger percentage of one-year-olds died of tuberculosis, compared to those under one year of age. As early as one year of age, deaths by tuberculosis was on the rise. The older children became, the more susceptible they became to the deadly disease. Of the one-year-olds who died from tuberculosis, 6 (40 percent) were males and 9 (60 percent) were females, a gender trend that would be maintained throughout most of the twentieth century. This gender split between deaths of males and females continued into adulthood, as more females died of tuberculosis than males. The fact that more females than males died of tuberculosis may be biological, but it may also be tied to social patterns and gender roles. Within Yakama families, females served as the primary caretakers of the infirm. Of course, this does not account for infant and childhood deaths caused by pneumonia which killed more males than females. However, the fact that females were primary caretakers may provide some insight into the deaths of females among adolescents and young adults. Indeed, in Yakama society, females in general spent more time than males working within the home, particularly if someone became ill. Females were expected to care for the family members stricken with disease which put females at greater risk than males of being exposed to tuberculosis and other communicable diseases. However, males died more often of pneumonia, but most of these deaths occurred while they were infants and small children. Females experienced long term exposure to tuberculosis within the home, and they spent more time with those members of the family who had contracted the disease. Still, even among children one year of age females died more often than males from tuberculosis.

Miscellaneous accidents took the lives of 8 (6 percent) children one year of age (figure 3.7). Of those children one year of age who died from miscellaneous accidents, 6 (75 percent) were males and 2 (25 percent) were females. Males were more likely to die of accidental deaths than females, perhaps because of their type of play. Small children generally imitated the lives of their parents. Both boys and girls occasionally played in dangerous places where their lives could be placed in jeopardy, particularly by drowning. More children died of drowning than of any other accidental cause. One Yakama child one year of age died after being struck by a train, while two died from suffocation when their homes burned to the ground. In a few cases, the Death Certificates are specific, one stating that a child had drowned while playing. In other cases, the records are not revealing about details involving accidents suffered by boys and girls. Clearly, the older children became, the more susceptible they were to death by accidents. Miscellaneous accidents did not occur in the age group under one year of age, but it became an important cause of death among children one year of age and older. Deaths caused by miscellaneous accidents were a marked cause of death among Yakama of all ages from one year of age to ninety-nine. The more active and mobile people became, the more they ran the risk of dying by accidental causes.

Among one-year-olds, whooping cough followed miscellaneous accidents as the fifth leading cause of death (figure 3.7). Whooping cough took the lives of 7 (5 percent) children one year of age. Like miscellaneous accidents, whooping cough was not a major cause of death among children under one year of age. However, whooping cough was the cause of death of a sufficient number of Yakama children to warrant note. Of the Yakama children who died of whooping cough, 4 (57 percent) were males and 3 (43 percent) were females, a fairly even split between the two sexes. Among children one year of age, the largest number to die in any one year died in 1918. A total of 23 children died that year when Spanish influenza swept across the Northwest, but only 1 child one year of age died of influenza that year, while 5 died of pneumonia which probably was affected by influenza. Thus, influenza may have influenced the large number of deaths suffered by one-year-olds in 1918, and it was likely a contributing or underlying factor of other causes of death.

Summary

Overall, the largest concentration of deaths among one-year-olds occurred between 1910 and 1926 with a peak year of death in 1918. The influenza epidemic probably weakened the resistance of one-year-olds, allowing other diseases, including pneumonia, gastrointestinal disorders, and tuberculosis to prey upon small children. Another concentration of deaths in this age category occurred between 1924 and 1945. From 1945 through 1964, the statistics show a gradual decline in the number of deaths of one-year-old children, which seems to be the result of improved public health, sanitation, antibiotics, and medical health care on the Yakama Reservation. In any case, children one year of age suffered the second largest number of deaths experienced by any age group on the Yakama Reservation from 1888 to 1964, and these deaths were caused by pneumonia, gastrointestinal disorders, tuberculosis, miscellaneous accidents, and whooping cough.

Yakama Children under Six but More Than Two Years of Age

Children under six but more than two years of age also suffered great loss of life between 1888 and 1964. The number of deaths of Yakama children ages two, three, four, and five declined with each successive year, but these age groups experienced more deaths than any other age from six through ninety-nine. A total of 276 (7 percent) children under six but more than two years of age died on the Yakama Reservation. Children were less likely to die the longer they lived and the closer they were to five years of age. However, their journey from birth through age five was a perilous one. A total of 112 Yakama children two years of age and 67 children three years of age died during the era from 1888 to 1964. Among children four years of age, 62 deaths occurred, and children five years of age suffered 35 deaths during the seventy-six-year period under examination. Of the 276 children mentioned above, 126 (46 percent) were males and 149 (53 percent) were females (the gender of one child was unrecorded). In comparison to Yakama children in the age groups of under one year of age and one year of age, more females than males died in that age category of under six but more than two.

Pneumonia was the foremost killer of children under six but more than two years of age, taking the lives of 70 (41 percent) children (figure 3.8). Pneumonia was the leading killer of Yakama children in all three categories, and it remained an important cause of death as children got older. The percentage of deaths caused by pneumonia was slightly less than for children one year of age, but pneumonia remained a significant cause of death. Of the Yakama children under six and more than two years of age who died of pneumonia, 37 (53 percent) were males and 33 (47 percent) were females, indicating that about an even number of males and females died of the dreaded disease in this age category.

Tuberculosis was the second most dangerous cause of death among Yakama children under six but more than two years of age (figure 3.8). A total of 33 (19 percent) children died of tuberculosis, and of these children under six but more than two years of age, 13 (39 percent) were males and 20 (61 percent) were females. As was the case with children one year of age and within the general population of Yakama people, females died more often from tuberculosis than males. Yakama children were exposed to the tubercle bacilli in their homes, schools, and churches. Nearly everyone living on or near the Yakama Reservation had friends and relatives with the disease, and none of the people could avoid breathing the air that contained deadly bacilli. Tuberculosis was an indiscriminate killer of young and old alike, but it thrived in Yakama children the older they became, particularly in children in their late teenage years.

Gastrointestinal disorders continued to plague children after the age of two, and it was the third most common cause of death in children under six but more than two years of age (figure 3.8). Among children in this age group, 15 (9 percent) died of gastrointestinal disorders. Of those children who died of disorders of the stomach, intestines, and digestive tract, 10 (67 percent) were males and 5 (33 percent) were females. Although the number of deaths by gastrointestinal disorders declined as children got older, the condition remained a significant killer. Children eating new foods and drinking impure liquids sometimes invited deadly bacilli into their digestive systems. They also contracted influenza viruses that infected their digestive tract, causing vomiting, diarrhea, and dehydration. Disorders involving the stomach, intestines, and colon were a major cause of death among Yakama children, and 85 percent of all gastrointestinal–related deaths experienced by Yakama people from 1888 to 1964 were deaths that occurred in the age group under five.

Meningitis is an infection of three membranes surrounding the brain, and between 1888 and 1964, a total of 13 (8 percent) Yakama children who were under six but more than two years of age died of meningitis (figure 3.8). Of the children dying of meningitis, 9 (69 percent) were males and 4 (31 percent) were females. Male children on the Yakama Reservation were more likely to die from meningitis than females. Meningitis was followed in importance by miscellaneous accidents as a cause of death among Yakama children under six but more than two years of age. Miscellaneous accidents included severe burns from a grassfire and house fire, gunshot wound, barbiturate poisoning, three drownings, and an "alleged fall." Miscellaneous accidents was the fifth most common cause of death for Yakama children in this age group. A total of 9 (5 percent) children lost their lives through miscellaneous accidents not related to automobiles. Of those children dying as a result of miscellaneous accidents, 4 (44 percent) were males and 5 (56 percent) were females. This represents a fairly even split between males and females, but the figures indicate that a change had occurred. In the previous age group of one year olds, boys were more likely to die as a result of miscellaneous accidents by a three to one margin. As females became older and more active, they became more adventuresome, traveling into situations that were potentially dangerous. As a result, miscellaneous accidents among females grew more frequent and fatal.

The largest number of deaths in the age group of under six but more than two years of age occurred in 1930 when 37 children died. The heaviest concentration of deaths for children of this age group was between 1926 and 1931 when 115 (42 percent) children died. During the era from 1888 to 1964, the five leading causes of death among children under six but more than two years of age were pneumonia, tuberculosis, gastrointestinal disorders, meningitis, and miscellaneous accidents.

Analysis

Death Certificates of the Yakama Indian Agency provide a glimpse into one aspect of Yakama Indian history, and they are clear on a few points regarding the known causes of deaths among children. Most important, the largest concentration of deaths among Yakama Indians of all ages from birth to ninety-nine was among children under six years of age. Among all Yakama, the modal age group was that of Yakama infants under one year of age. The second largest number of deaths occurred among children one year of age, and the third largest number of deaths occurred in that group of children under six but more than two years of age. Collectively, deaths of Yakama children (including fetal deaths) under six years of age constitute a total of 737 (33 percent) deaths between the years of 1888 to 1964.

In all three age categories of Yakama children, the leading cause of death was pneumonia, and the effects of this disease remained constant in terms of its percentages within each of the three age groups (figure 4.8). Furthermore, the ill effects of gastrointestinal disorders also remained constant among all three age groups. By contrast, tuberculosis became a more important cause of death the older the child became, moving from 3 percent of all childhood deaths for those Yakama under one year of age to 11 percent for one-year-olds to 19 percent for children under six but more than two years of age. However, tuberculosis caused the most deaths among Yakama teen-agers and people in their twenties. A total of 43 percent of all tuberculosis deaths suffered by Yakama people struck the age group of 15-29. Although tuberculosis was a notable cause of death among all children, it was a greater killer of children in their late teens as well as young adults.

While heart disease and syphilis were leading causes of death among children under one year of age, these causes of death did not appear in the other two age categories for Yakama children. This is likely because these diseases resulted from problems originating while the child was in utero. On the other hand, while whooping cough appears as a marked cause of death among Yakama children one year of age and was the sixth most important cause of death among children under six but more than two years of age, it was not a major cause of death among children under one year of age. Meningitis appeared as a major cause of death only among children under six but more than two years of age. Miscellaneous accidents were not an important cause of death among infants less than one year of age, but they became an increasingly significant cause of death among children after their first birthday. Indeed, miscellaneous accidents ranked fourth among the ten leading causes of death within the general Yakama population from 1888 to 1964.

Premature births and stillbirths occurred often on the Yakama Reservation, and prematurity ranked ninth overall as a cause of death within the general Yakama population. Furthermore, among all causes of death experienced by males during the seventy-six year period covered by the study, premature births ranked eighth as a cause of death. Most likely, many premature births and stillbirths were importantly influenced by poverty and inadequate medical care, particularly prenatal care. In large measure, Yakama people as a whole and children in particular suffered from what Yakama call "white man's disease" because of the lack of prenatal care, preventive medicine, and prescription drugs. The government of the United States did not sufficiently fund the Office of Indian Affairs so that the health division of the bureau could protect the lives of Yakama children. Clearly, the government broke its treaty obligation with Yakama people when it failed to provide adequate health care. However, it is worth noting that inadequate health care was not primarily the fault of health care providers on the Yakama Reservation, for some of these men and women tried to better health care for Yakama people. Lack of funding for health personnel, staff development, new medicines, health education programs, and hospital-clinic-sanitarium facilities was the impediment to quality health care, not generally the commitment of nurses, doctors, and field matrons.

Although the primary causes of death for Yakama children were diseases brought to the area through white contact, the underlying cause of death was poverty. The substandard living condition among Yakama people was the result of American Indian policies, the reservation system, white settlement, malnutrition, settled lifestyle, unsanitary dwellings, and overcrowded housing. The government of the United States forced the Yakama onto a reservation, where public health and sanitation were nearly nonexistent for much of the twentieth century, and it supported the destruction of natural food sources by encouraging white settlement of the inland Northwest. White farmers and ranchers limited access of Native Americans to their natural food sources, and they destroyed the plants and animals of the region that provided food for Yakama.

Farmers and ranchers joined forces with the government to dam the rivers and divert water for electrical power and irrigation. This destroyed salmon runs, so vital to the livelihood and spiritual well-being of Yakama people. Lumber companies harmed animal habitats in the forests of the western boundary of the reservation. Agents of the Office of Indian Affairs supported an end to the seasonal rounds followed by the Yakama in order to "civilize" and Christianize Indians through new settlement patterns that promoted agriculture and ranching. The results of white settlement and government policies were nothing less than extreme poverty and destructive diseases. Death came to the Yakama during the late nineteenth and early twentieth centuries, claiming the lives of numerous members of the Yakama Nation. Death indiscriminately seized men and women, boys and girls, taking the lives of hundreds of fetuses, infants, toddlers, and small children.

Cause of Death and Gender

Between 1888 and 1964, a total of 2,827 Death Certificates indicated a known cause of death. The ten most frequent causes of death were scrutinized to determine the number and percent of males and females that died from each of the major causes. An examination of this data is instructive (figure 3.11). As has been established, the foremost cause of death on the Yakama Reservation was tuberculosis, and more women died of the disease than men. Of the 619 people who died of tuberculosis, 329 (54 percent) were females and 289 (46 percent) were males. Although linked to biological factors, this was likely influenced by the fact that women worked within the home and were primary caretakers of ill members of their families. However, this female/male differential is a common trend within populations around the world, and it may be tied more exclusively to biological factors.[76] In the case of pneumonia, 323 (57 percent) males died of the disease while 242 (43 percent) women succumbed to pneumonia. The difference in the numbers is the result of the deaths from pneumonia suffered by male babies, since pneumonia was the leading killer of all children less than six years of age, particularly males. Women may have died more often of tuberculosis than of pneumonia because individuals were more likely to contract tuberculosis the older they became. Women caring for ill patients suffering from tuberculosis were generally exposed to the disease for a longer period of time as it developed among members of their families.

A total of 322 Yakama people died of heart diseases during the seventy-six-year period. Of these, 164 (52 percent) were women and 158 (48 percent) were men, a fairly even split between males and females. Miscellaneous accidents caused the death of far more men than women. Between 1888 and 1964, 114 (79 percent) Yakama men died by accidents, while only 31 (21 percent) women died as a result of them. Men probably died of miscellaneous accidents more often than women because they worked outside the home more often than women. This is not to suggest that women living on the Yakama Reservation did not work outside the home, because they did. Some Yakama women worked as migrant laborers and usually maintained their own family's farm or ranch. Thus, some women worked for wages as did men.

That women also farmed and ranched their family's lands is evidenced by the large number and types of purchases Yakama women made. Between 1909 and 1912. For example, women made more purchases than men of horses, cattle, wagons, buggies, hacks, and miscellaneous home-ranch supplies and tools. Moreover, women also spent more money on purchases than did men during the same time period.[77] The evidence suggests that women were deeply involved in the economic lives of their families and that men working outside the home died more often than women of accidents. Yakama men worked at a variety of jobs relating to farming, fishing, logging, and ranching. Some of them died from accidents resulting from "grass fires," or from having been "drowned while fishing," "thrown from a horse," or "crushed by falling logs." During the early twentieth century, Yakama men spent more time away from home doing day labor, and they were more prone to accidents. The result is a larger number of accidental deaths among Yakama men than Yakama women.[78]

As has been indicated, another important cause of death on the reservation was gastrointestinal disorders. A total of 124 Yakama people died of gastrointestinal disorders, 65 (52 percent) of whom were females and 59 (48 percent) males. This is nearly an even division of deaths experienced by females and males, and this nearly-equal division between the sexes is also the case with deaths caused by automobile accidents. However, slightly more males died as a result of automobile accidents than did females. A total of 122 Yakama died in car accidents between 1924, when the first accident occurred, and 1964. Of these people, 71 (58 percent) were men and 51 (42 percent) were women. More men than women died in automobile accidents probably because men used family vehicles to travel to and from work and took more trips to border towns. In addition, males died slightly more often than females as a result of the consumption of alcohol. Mixing alcohol and driving accounts for some male deaths.

A few more females than males died of influenza during the seventy-six year period. A total of 104 people died of different varieties of influenza, 58 (56 percent) of whom were females and 46 (44 percent) males. The fact that females died of the disease more often than males may be tied to biological factors, but, as with tuberculosis, that females were also primary caretakers within the family, making them more likely to be exposed to high concentrations of various bacteria and viruses. Yakama lived in small, enclosed houses where individuals were in close proximity with each other, sharing the air they breathed and common eating and cooking utensils. Females also died more often than did males from cancer, and they were particularly susceptible to uterine, cervical, breast, and stomach cancers. A total of 82 Yakama died of cancer between 1888 and 1964. Of these, 58 (71 percent) were females and 24 (29 percent) were males. A total of 44 women died of uterine, stomach, breast, and cervical cancer (in order of their importance), and these were the four leading causes of cancer among females (figure 4.6). Together, they contributed to 76 percent of all cancer experienced by women. Stomach and prostate–rectal cancers were the leading causes of cancer deaths suffered by Yakama males. From 1925 to 1964, lung cancer killed only five individuals, including two women and three men. During this time period, only two Yakama, a male forty years old and a female nine years old, died of leukemia. Lung cancer and leukemia were not prominent causes of death among the Yakama during the early twentieth century, but their importance as causes of death may have increased after the 1960s due to tobacco use and the location of Hanford Nuclear Plant near the border of the Yakama Reservation. The effects of tobacco use and the Hanford Nuclear Plant in terms of cancer deaths and other causes of death have yet to be explored by scholars.[79] Yakama depended on water downstream from the plant, drinking water and eating fish taken from the river.

More males than females died as a result of premature births on the Yakama Reservation, a circumstance that is common in other populations of the world (figures 3.5, 3.10). Female babies tend to be more hardy than males, and thus males die more frequently than females. On the Yakama Reservation, a total of 64 fetuses died as a consequence of premature birth, of whom 38 (59 percent) were males and 26 (41 percent) females. However, a few more females died of senility than men. Of the 57 Yakama who died of senility and old age, 31 (54 percent) were women while 26 (46 percent) were men.

Comparison of Causes of Death among Females and Males

An examination of the ten leading causes of death of women and of men demonstrates that some differences occur in the importance of specific diseases among people of different gender. The discussion is based on known causes of death among males and females. Among the 1,927 females that died between 1888 and 1964, the cause of death is known for 1,352 (70 percent) of them. Of the 1,960 males that died during the same era, the cause of death of 1,458 (74 percent) is known. Although tuberculosis and pneumonia were the two leading causes of death within the general Yakama population, tuberculosis was the foremost cause of death among females, accounting for 329 (24 percent) deaths. By contrast, pneumonia was the leading cause of death among males, accounting for 323 (22 percent) deaths (figure 3.11). Pneumonia was the second most important cause of death among females, while tuberculosis was the second leading cause of death among males.

Heart disease was the third leading cause of death among Yakama females and males, but miscellaneous accidents ranked fourth as a cause of death among males, while miscellaneous accidents were not among the top ten causes of death among Yakama females. Gastrointestinal disorders ranked fourth among Yakama females as a cause of death. Males died from both of these causes because of travel to and from work and because of the hazardous nature of the work place (most often associated with farming and ranching). Males also died more often from automobile accidents than did women. Like miscellaneous accidents, automobile accidents did not rank among the top ten causes of death among Yakama females. Moreover, males died more often as a result of premature births than did females. Premature birth was the eighth leading causes of death among males, while it was far less important as a cause of death among Yakama females. In addition, a total of 28 (2 percent) Yakama men suffered alcohol-related deaths of all kinds, while this cause of death was not a marked cause of death for Yakama females.

Females died more often than males of cancer, meningitis, and influenza. These three causes of death ranked fifth as causes of death among females on the Yakama Reservation. A total of 58 (4 percent) females died of each of these diseases. Females suffered significantly from cancer, and females experienced 71 percent of all cancer-related deaths on the reservation. Nearly all of the cancer deaths (76 percent) among females on the Yakama Reservation were from cancer of the uterus, stomach, breasts, and cervix. While cancer was the fifth leading cause of death among Yakama females, it ranked tenth among Yakama males. Females also experienced 58 deaths as a result of meningitis and 58 deaths as a result of influenza. The Death Certificates indicate that Yakama men and women died of tubercular meningitis as well as other forms that attacked the brain.

Meningitis was responsible for several deaths among Yakama children, particularly females. This cause does not appear in the ten leading causes of death among Yakama males, but it was as important as influenza and cancer among Yakama females. This is also the case for strokes, natural causes, and childbirths—causes of death among Yakama females not found in the foremost causes of death among Yakama males. A total of 30 (2 percent) women died of strokes, 24 (2 percent) died of natural causes, and 23 (2 percent) died while in childbirth (figure 3.11). The number of females dying in childbirth is another indication of poor health care, inadequate health facilities, and the lack of health education programs. Abdel Omran has pointed out that some women develop rickets in their youth, causing pelvic deformities that complicate childbirth and cause higher rates of maternal death.[80] This factor may have contributed to maternal deaths among Yakama women, but without autopsies and medical explanations of death, it is impossible to determine from Yakama Death Certificates what role rickets played in the deaths of mothers during childbirth.

Conclusion

Overall, males and females shared the most serious causes of death, including tuberculosis, pneumonia, and heart disease. But there were some marked differences in causes of death between the sexes. Males died more often from accidental deaths and automobile accidents. They also suffered alcohol-related deaths, although alcohol was not as important of a cause of death among Yakama people as it has been in more recent years. Some individuals stereotype Indians regarding alcohol, but from 1888 through 1964, Yakamas suffered relatively few alcohol-related deaths. Still, 51 people died of alcohol-related deaths during the seventy-six year period of this study, including males and females who died of alcohol poisoning, liver failure, or alcoholism. Of these deaths, 23 (48 percent) were females and 28 (55 percent) were males. While a larger number of males than females died of alcohol, far more Yakama females died of cancer and meningitis.

Finally, males and females also died in fairly equal numbers as victims of murders and suicides. A total of 23 Yakama people died as a result of murders during the era from 1888 to 1964. Of these, 11 males and 12 females met violent deaths by murder. In addition, a total of 17 Yakama died by suicide, including 8 females and 9 males. A person's gender did not seem to influence the number of deaths resulting from murder and suicide. However, in some specific cases, gender was an important factor in the cause of death suffered by Yakama males and females, and it is illuminating to view the similarities and differences in the causes of death on the Yakama Reservation.

Notes

1. "Tuberculosis Among North American Indians," 55–72.

2. Carr to Commissioner of Indian Affairs, 17 June 1917 and Sprague to Carr, 5 May 1917, "Health & Hospitalization Records and Reports, 1912–1940," Yakama Agency, Box 264, NA, PNWR, RG 75. Some of the general works regarding tuberculosis include Michael E. Teller, *The Tuberculosis Movement: A Public Health Campaign in the Progressive Era* (New York: Greenwood Press, 1988); Waksman, *The Conquest of Tuberculosis*; and Smith, *The Retreat of Tuberculosis, 1850–1950*.

3. Dubos and Dubos, *The White Plague*, 189.

4. Ibid., xix, 69, 94, 100–10, 115.

5. Ibid., 115–16.

6. Ibid., 4.

7. Ibid., 117–19.

8. Ibid., 120–21.

9. Ibid., 127–28.

10. As quoted in Ibid., 127. Dubos and Dobos provide an excellent discussion of one's state of mind and disease, see 148–53. Also, see Smith, *The Retreat of Tuberculosis, 1850–1950*, 27.

11. Dubos and Dubos, *The White Plague*, 191.

12. Boyd, "The Introduction of Infectious Diseases Among the Indians of the Pacific Northwet, 1774–1874," 344–61, 488, 524–25.

13. Dubos and Dubos, *The White Plague*, 170–72, 218–19, 227; Preston and Haines, *Fatal Years*, 209.

14. Dubos and Dubos, *The White Plague*, 140, 142, 174–75, 198–99, 203, 206; Smith, *The Retreat of Tuberculosis, 1850–1950*, 5, 8–11, 13, 19.

15. Indian Health Service, "Trends in Indian Health—1991" (Washington, D.C.: United States Department of Health and

Human Services, 1991), 4 (hereafter cited as IHS, "Trends in Indian Health").

16. Popkin, "Nutritional Patterns and Transitions," 138-39.

17. Hunn, *Nch'i-Wana*, 138-200, 282-84.

18. The statistics for African Americans and white Americans are from the United States Department of Commerce, *The Social and Economic Status of the Black Population in the United States: An Historical View, 1790-1978* (Washington, D.C.: United States Department of Commerce, 1978), 124-25 (hereafter cited as *Black Population*). The statistics for the general population of the United States are found in *Historical Statistics of the United States: Colonial Times to 1970* (Washington, D.C.: United States Department of Commerce, 1975), 58 (hereafter cited as *Historical Statistics*). For an excellent discussion linking American Indian poverty and health, see Carruth J. Wagner and Erwin S. Rabeau, "Indian Poverty and Indian Health," *United States Department of Health, Education, and Welfare Indicators* (March 1994): xxiv-xliv.

19. Ibid.; Dubos and Dubos, *The White Plague*, 185-87.

20. Ibid. All of the statistical sources mentioned in note 18 above and the book by the Dubos are pertinent to this discussion.

21. Oral interview by Clifford E. Trafzer with Brad Richie, M.D., 18 May 1993, Colton, California.

22. *Black Population*, 124.

23. Ibid., 124-25. The author makes the comparison here with the general population of the United States because the two diseases, pneumonia and influenza, were combined in *Historical Statistics*, 58.

24. *Black Population*, 124-25.

25. Ibid.; *Historical Statistics*, 58. In an article in *Circulation*, the journal of the American Heart Association (December 1996), William Eaton and a team of medical researchers at Johns Hopkins University point out that depression is a primary sources of stress and that it affects the risk of heart attack. Anomie among the Yakama and other Indian groups may well have contributed to increased rates of h eart disease and other illness that lead to death.

26. Only one Yakama died of heart disease in 1920 with a death rate of 34. In 1940, the Yakama death rate per 100,000 in the population was 224 and 171 in 1960. No information is available for 1910.

27. See the theoretical progression of dietary change in Popkin, "Nutritional Patterns and Tansitions," 139.

28. *Black Population*, 124–25; *Historical Statistics*, 58.

29. Ibid.

30. *Historical Statistics*, 58.

31. Yakama Death Certificates, NA, PNWR, RG 75.

32. Carr to Commissioner of Indian Affairs, 4 November 1918, "Medicine Man File," Yakama Agency, NA, PNWR, RG 75.

33. *Black Population*, 124–25.

34. Popkin, "Nutritional Patterns and Transitions," 138–40, 142–44.

35. Ibid.; *Historical Statistics*, 58.

36. *Black Population*, 124–25; *Historical Statistics*, 58.

37. For an entire scholarly study devoted to disease during this era, see Boyd, "The Introduction of Infectious Diseases Among Indians of the Pacific Northwest, 1774–1874."

38. Trafzer and Scheuerman, *Renegade Tribe*, 93–102; Hunn, *Nch'i-Wana*, 138–200; Schuster, "Yakima Indian Traditionalism," 243–46, 249–51. For an historical perspective of the importance of disease, see Alfred W. Crosby, *The Columbian Exchange: The Biological and Cultural Consequences of 1492* (Westport: Greenwood Publishing Co., 1972); Frederick Fox Cartwright, *Disease and History* (London: Hart-Davis, 1972); Howard Simpson, *Invisible Armies* (Indianapolis: Bobbs-Merrill, 1980); and Ann F. Ramenofsky, *Vectors of Death* (Albuquerque: University of New Mexico Press, 1987).

39. Kunz and Finkle, *Family Medical Guide*, 643–48; Trevathan, *Human Birth*, 12, 21, 67, 93, 98, 119, 124–125, 141–42, 199, 228.

40. Kunz and Finkle, *Family Medical Guide*, 643–48.

41. Ibid., 645.

42. Ibid., 647; Yakama Death Certificates, NA, PNWR, RG 75, Cases 699, 878, 3206, 4381, 2877, 2878.

43. Clayman, ed., *Encyclopedia of Medicine*, 941.

44. Trevathan, *Human Birth*, 11–12, 21, 75, 105, 142; Kunz and Finkle, *Family Medical Guide*, 647.

45. Yakama Death Certificates, NA, PNWR, RG 75, Cases 4525, 4327, 4553, 4991, 3930, 731, and 2908.

46. Spink, *Infectious Diseases*, 209–12; Burnet and White, *Natural History of Infectious Diseases*, 32–43, 52–69; Christie, *Infectious Diseases*, 269–99; and Kunz and Finkle, *Family Medical Guide*, 365, 695.

47. Kunz and Finkle, *Family Medical Guide*, 467, 664, 702; Christie, *Infectious Diseases*, 122–67; Spink, *Infectious Diseases*, 246–47; Burnet and White, *Natural History of Infectious Diseases*, 70–87.

48. Tuberculosis was the leading killer of all Yakama, ages 0–99, during the era from 1888 to 1964. See Hrdlickas, "Tuberculosis Among Certain Indian Tribes in the United States," 31–32; Spink, *Infectious Diseases*, 220–21, 224; Burnet and White, *Natural History of Infectious Diseases*, 213–24; Meyers, *Captain of All These Men of Death*, 73–83, 142–58; Waksman, *The Conquest of Tuberculosis*, 24.

49. Dubos and Dubos, *The White Plague*, 111–14; Smith, *The Retreat of Tuberculosis, 1850–1950*, 2–5.

50. Kunz and Finkle, *Family Medical Guide*, 574, 719, 748; Spink, *Infectious Diseases*, 220–22.

51. *San Bernardino Sun*, 15 March 1994, 15.

52. Waksman, *The Conquest of Tuberculosis*, 24; Meriam, *The Problem of Indian Administration*, 204–8.

53. Automobile accidents appeared as the seventh leading cause of death in the age group from two through five, but it was more important as the cause of death among the Yakama population over six years of age. Between 1888 and 1964, 121 Yakama died in car accidents, representing 3 percent of all deaths regardless of age.

54. Yakama Death Certificates, NA, PNWR, RG 75, Cases 4563, 4612, 4488, 3871, 4521.

55. Ramenofsky, *Vectors of Death*, 150–52; Kunz and Finkle, *Family Medical Guide*, 717. For two older works, specifically on whooping cough, see Joseph H. Lapin, *Whooping Cough* (Springfield, Ill.:

C. C. Thomas, 1943) and United States Public Health Service, *Whooping Cough* (Washington, D.C.: United States Public Health Service, 1957).

56. Recently meningitis emerged as a major killer in Mankato, Minnesota, killing young people, particularly those in their teens. See the front page of the *Los Angeles Times*, 7-8 May 1995.

57. Christie, *Infectious Diseases*, 619-71; Spink, *Infectious Diseases*, 295-97, 287-88, 290-94. For a recent medical study of meningitis, see J. D. Williams and J. Burnie, eds., *Bacterial Meningitis* (London: Academic Press, 1987).

58. Automobile deaths caused several deaths after the age of six.

59. Kunz and Finkle, *Family Medical Guide*, 663. According to the Indian Health Service, between 1987 and 1989, Sudden Infant Death Syndrome was the leading cause of infant death in the Portland area which includes the Yakama Reservation. It is an important cause of death today and was historically. See *Regional Differences in Indian Health* (Washington, D.C.: United States Department of Health and Human Services, 1993), 40.

60. Ibid., 671-72.

61. Trafzer and Scheuerman, *Renegade Tribe*, 25-26, 103-8.

62. Omran, "Epidemiologic Transition in the United States," 16-18.

63. Popkin, "Nutritional Patterns and Transitions," 138-40, 142-43, 153-54.

64. John R. Weeks, *Population: An Introduction to Concepts and Issues* (Belmont, California: Wadsworth Publishing Co., 1992), 177-78.

65. Firth to Trafzer, 1 December 1992, author's collection. According to Firth, "about 1% more males than females are born; males do die more easily."

66. Benson, "Race, Health, and Power," 6-20.

67. Ibid., 12-13; Car to Commissioner of Indian Affairs, 7 June 1917, "Health & Hospitalization Records and Reports, 1912-1940," Yakama Agency, Box 264, NA, PNWR, RG 75.

68. Carr to Commissioner of Indian Affairs, 7 June 1917, "Health & Hospitalization Records and Reports, 1912-1940," Yakama Agency, Box 264, NA, PNWR, RG 75.

69. Schuster, "Yakima Indian Traditionalism," 176-77.

70. Gregory R. Campbell, "The Political Epidemiology of Infant Mortality: A Health Crisis Among Montana American Indians," *American Indian Culture and Research Journal* 13 (1989): 106–8, 112–16.

71. Dubos and Dubos, *The White Plague*, 126.

72. Preston and Haines, *Fatal Years*, xix.

73. Ibid.

74. Benson, "Race, Health, and Power," 278–82.

75. Ibid., 301–17.

76. The cause of death for 93 people was unknown.

77. A total of 106 deaths were unknown, while 170 were known.

78. Dubos and Dubos, *The White Plague*, 126.

79. Clifford E. Trafzer, "Horses and Cattle, Buggies and Hacks: Purchases by Yakima Indian Women, 1909–1912," in Nancy Shoemaker, ed., *Negotiators of Change: Historical Perspectives on Native American Women* (New York: Routledge, 1995), 176–92.

80. Yakama Death Certificates, NA, PNWR. RG 75, Cases 3338, 1314, 70, 3972.

81. Oral communication, author with John Moran, M.D., Indian Health Service, Yakama Reservation, 4 May 1993. Also see John Moran, Yakama Indian Health Center Morbidity and Mortality Committee, "1991 Mortality Report," 19 November 1992, Yakama Indian Health Center, Toppenish, Washington, Yakama Reservation. For a study of women and their contact with non-Indians in terms of trade, see Trafzer, "Horses, Cattle, Buggies, and Hacks," 176–92.

82. Omran, "Epidemiologic Transition in the United States," 17.

Part Five

CONCLUSION

Yakama Reservation underwent major epidemiological and nutritional transitions over time. They have survived radical cultural changes, the difficulties of a white invasion of their lands, and the trials that ensued after the imposition of the Yakama Treaty of 1855. The harvest of the American invasion and that agreement led to what has been called the Plateau Indian War of 1855-58 and the establishment of the reservation system in the Pacific Northwest. In turn, the reservation system exacerbated the effects of infectious diseases that spread throughout the Northwest during the Age of Pestilence, beginning in the late eighteenth and early nineteenth centuries.

Although most whites intended reservations to be places where the United States could "civilize" and Christianize Indians, the Yakama reservation, like most, became a host to disease and social-cultural circumstances that led to foreshortened lives and high death rates among its population. During the nineteenth century, the Yakama fell victim to a rash of diseases that persisted well into the late twentieth century.

Unfortunately, we do not presently have statistical information from Death Certificates for this era, and it is not until the early twentieth century that this data is in sufficient quality and quantity to assess deaths on the Yakama Reservation. Still, Yakama people survived the Age of Pestilence and rebounded during the Age of Receding Pandemics.[1]

Although the Yakama population grew in the twentieth century, its death rates continued to be elevated. There is no question that death continued to stalk the Yakama in the first four decades of the twentieth century; this work is a first assessment of Yakama clinical death based on the best documentary information available, Death Certificates.

The government of the United States forced the Yakama and thirteen other distinct tribes and bands onto the Yakama Reservation, designating them in most documents, including Death Certificates, as generic "Yakama Indians." Although incorrect, this description was used throughout the work to describe all native peoples living on the Yakama Reservation, because in using Death Certificates, Death Registers, and Birth Registers, there was no way to distinguish among Palouse, Wishram, or Klickitat, since they were nearly always labeled "Yakama" by recording agents of the county and state.

On the Yakama Reservation, the Office of Indian Affairs ruled over all of these Indians through Indian agents who were charged with caring for the people. This included overseeing health care provided the people, a task which some officials attempted to accomplish in spite of inadequate funding from the United States government. Throughout the late nineteenth and early twentieth centuries, the Yakama Agency lacked public health programs, the means to improve sanitation, medical personnel, advanced medicines, and hospitals–clinics. Unfortunately, employees of the Office of Indian Affairs— agents, doctors, nurses—failed miserably at their task of providing quality health care primarily because of the lack of resources. Yakama men, women, and children perished as a result. The Congress of the United States and the Office of Indian Affairs bear much of the responsibility for poor health care because of the lack of funding for Indian health programs.

The reservation system changed many aspects of Native American life, and Indian agents controlled nearly every aspect of that life. Through instructions from the Office of Indian

Affairs, Yakama agents sought to destroy two elements of traditional life among Plateau Indians. First, agents altered the traditional pattern of seasonal rounds among the people, so that they could not travel about the Plateau gathering roots and berries, hunting deer and antelope, and fishing salmon and sturgeon. Policies of the United States government directed agents to force Indians to remain on the reservation, farming and ranching so that whites could "civilize" the people. This circumstance led to many changes detrimental to Yakama people, including dietary and housing changes that promoted poor hygiene on the reservation. Second, agents actively sought to destroy native culture, particularly Indian religions, such as the *Wáshat*, Shaker Church, and *Waptashi* (Feather Religion). Destruction or interruption of native religions, officials reasoned, would aid in the Christianization and "civilization" of Indians. This was national Indian policy, and the significance of these policies in terms of Indian health is immeasurable (figure 4.4).

These developments were detrimental to the physical, mental, and spiritual well-being of Native Americans living on the Yakama Reservation. Forcing Yakama people to live settled lives prevented them from eating traditional and nutritious foods. Forcing them to remain on the reservation fostered new types of housing that were injurious to their health. Rather than living in temporary mat lodges and tipis and moving from place to place, Yakama people lived in small, unventilated wooden shacks conducive to the spread and proliferation of dangerous viruses and bacilli that infected and killed men, women, and children at a high rate. The people lived in close quarters with each other without knowledge of public health, sanitation, and medical matters. Forcing the people to live on the Yakama Reservation gave Christians an opportunity to subvert native religions and convert native peoples to Euro-American religions. This created a cultural crisis within the reservation community between those people who continued to worship the Washat in the long house religion or through the Feather Religion and those who found Jesus and walked one of the many sectarian roads of Christianity—including the Indian Shaker Church which agents disliked. In the late nineteenth and early twentieth centuries, the Yakama experienced a social depression that harmed the larger Indian community. The reservation system created an unhealthy environment which encouraged viral and bacterial invasions of Yakama people that were as disastrous—or more so—as the political and military conquest they had suffered in the nineteenth century.

In order to monitor the health statistics of Indians on the reservations, in 1884, Congress ordered the Office of Indian Affairs to collect vital statistics regarding births and deaths. Although the Office of Indian Affairs did not require agents to prepare and preserve Death Certificates, the office expected agents to keep registers of births and deaths from which to derive a statistical base, and, later, to help county and state officials record deaths and births. This was a federal mandate in 1884, not a state or territorial law. Agents on the Yakama Reservation failed to collect death statistics until 1888, and, even then, they failed in their endeavor. In 1888, the Yakama Agency reported one death within a native population of 1,765 people. Although this is an unrealistic figure, this study begins with the first recorded death on the Yakama Reservation. For a variety of reasons, agents failed to collect vital statistics until 1910, although the most complete data on the reservation is that recorded by the county and state through Death Certificates after 1924. Washington state became a death registry state in 1907, but the Death Certificates collected by the agency between 1907 and 1923 are not numerous. Agents kept copies of these Death Certificates at the Yakama Agency, and these documents are the basis of this study. Between 1888 and 1910, Yakama agents recorded or collected only a few death documents, and the information found in these death records is incomplete and of little help. Still, they are included in the data because they are a part of the entire body of data base. These scant records do reflect the lack of interest on the part of the agents to collect and preserve vital statistics, even after their job was made easier in 1907 when Washington became a death registry state.

In 1924, agents on the Yakama Reservation began making a major effort to collect and keep copies of Death Certificates completed by the Yakama County Health Department on behalf of the state of Washington. Indians, agents, and employees of the Yakama Agency helped provide this data during the 1920s, in large part because of the national movement to examine and reform American Indian affairs. One of the central concerns of white reformers was Native American health, but they were hampered in their investigations because of the lack of data available on reservations regarding births and deaths. Clearly, in order for the government to assess the general health of Indian people, particularly in relation to specific diseases, health officials and policy makers needed accurate figures on the number of deaths, causes of death, age at death, place of death, sex of individuals, and other pieces of information. Complete information on these variables was not generally recorded until the 1920s (figures 1.1, 1.10).

Death data for the Yakama Agency provides historians new and detailed insights into the conditions of native peoples living and dying on one reservation during the first six decades of the twentieth century. Moreover, Death Certificates provide scholars with a new voice, one that has been largely ignored in the Native American past but that is critical in a study of American Indians. Statistical data offers a voice of common native people—men, women, and children—who left their mark through their act of birth and death. In this case, the record of their act of dying informs us about their age at death, gender, cause of death, place of death, and blood quantum. Death data provides a unique understanding of certain aspects of reservation life that heretofore have not been the subject of scholarly inquiry. In addition, data taken from the Death Certificates offers voices from different eras focusing on the causes of death among individual native populations. For example, although tuberculosis was the foremost cause of death among Yakama people from 1888 to 1964, health officials on the Yakama Reservation arrested the disease during the 1940s so that after that decade, it was an insignificant cause of death on the reservation.

The statistics generated from the Death Certificates are most helpful if one has an historical understanding of the Indians from the Columbia Plateau, particularly the Yakama. Before white contact, Indians of the Columbia Plateau believed that in addition to several common causes of death, there were three major explanations of malevolent deaths. They believed that spirit sickness, rattlesnake medicine, and witchcraft were all viable explanations of death within the culture, although these explanations of death may have been brought about through warfare, infections, or accidents. Thus, these spiritual causes of death were—and to some extent still are—significant, underlying causes of death and continued to be important culturally among the Yakama and their neighbors even after the arrival of whites. However, Indians recognized that the *suyapo* brought new forms of death that infected native communities, killing large numbers of people. Indians classified these new causes of death as "white man's diseases," and native peoples—elders and Indian doctors—could not control these new scourges with old remedies. These new causes of death are the only ones recorded on Death Registers and Death Certificates.

In a sense, there were two reservations or two distinct cultures on the reservation—one native and one white. These cultures coexisted and overlapped in some ways, but in many more ways they were distinct, different, and unique. Native culture recognized and feared various forms of spiritual sickness and the power of medicine people acknowledged the need for culturally prescribed traditions, medicines, foods, and behavior. The other culture was derived from a European background that discredited spiritual sickness as superstitious, backward, and akin to devil worship. No official for the Yakama County Coroner's Office, Health Department, or the Washington State Health Department ever recorded a "traditional" explanation of death during the seventy-six years under consideration in this study. The evidence indicates that agents knew of the native belief in non-Western causes of death, but never took these explanations of death seriously. Certainly, most Yakama agents learned of native beliefs about death and its causes, but they discounted them, which is not surprising given the cultural assumptions of white officials. Native American beliefs about causes of death were viewed by whites as superstitions, unworthy of note. However, traditional causes of death among Yakama and other Indians living on the reservation were and are valid explanations of death given native belief systems. Today, some Indians believe that traditional causes of death can manifest themselves through spirit sickness, witchcraft, or other negative power. These causes of death can also be used to foster accidents, suicides, pneumonia, heart disease, and other causes of death.

While it is important to recognize that the Yakama believe in traditional causes of death, it is difficult to assess the impact of these causes over time. Indeed, it is impossible to measure these causes. In contrast, Death Certificates created by whites provide a wealth of information about non-traditional causes of death among the sexes of different age groups over a lengthy period of time. The documents offer clinical explanations of death, not medical explanations. Still, they are instructive. The documents inform us about many causes of death, particularly tuberculosis, pneumonia, and heart disease, which were the three leading causes of death on the Yakama Reservation. Between 1888 and 1964, a total of 54 percent of all Yakama died of these three diseases. In order to put these deaths in perspective, the study offers a comparison of crude death rates resulting from specific causes of death among different populations in the United States.

Crude death rates are presented per 100,000 in the population, comparing a small population with large populations (figures 3.12, 4.4). These crude death rates are helpful in assessing the importance of each major cause of death within the Yakama population. For example, in 1930 and 1940, the Yakama had a crude death rate caused by tuberculosis that was many times greater than that of whites and African Americans. Even more dramatic is a comparison of the crude death rates resulting from pneumonia, a disease that thrived fairly unabated on the Yakama Reservation from 1888 to 1964. In 1930 and 1940, the Yakama had a crude death rate resulting from pneumonia that was many times greater than that of the African American population and more than twenty times greater than that of whites in the United States (figure 4.4). Although the crude death rate resulting from pneumonia among the Yakama decreased after the 1930s, it was still many times greater than that among other populations in the United States until 1964, particularly when compared to the white population. In addition, the Yakama experienced high crude death rates resulting from gastrointestinal disorders, automobile accidents, miscellaneous accidents, and premature births. They also had a high crude death rate caused by influenza, although most deaths from influenza occurred before 1930. Remarkably, full-blood Yakama people suffered 97 percent of all deaths resulting from influenza. These are illuminating findings, and Yakama voices speak to us through these statistics.

In addition to high crude death rates, the Yakama also suffered many fetal, infant, and childhood deaths (figures 1.6, 3.5,

3.6, 3.7, 3.8, 4.9, 4.10, 4.12). Fetal deaths and deaths of individuals less than six years of age constituted 33 percent of all
deaths on the reservation, with the modal age of death being
those children under one year of age. Premature births and
stillbirths were the two recorded causes of fetal deaths among
Yakama. In comparison to whites in the United States, Yakama
had a higher fetal death rate between 1926, when the best data
becomes available, and 1949. After 1949, the trend of fetal death
rates among the Yakama when compared to whites is also
erratic. In comparison to non–whites in the United States, the
Yakama fetal death rate is erratic between 1926 and 1944, with
the Yakama having the higher fetal death rate at times and the
non–white population experiencing a higher fetal death rate at
other times. After 1944, non–whites consistently experienced a
higher fetal death rate than did Yakama people. In comparison
to whites in the United States, the Yakama had a higher—
sometimes many times higher—infant mortality rate, except for
the year of 1948. This was generally true in comparisons of
Yakama infant mortality rates with those experienced over time
by the non–white population of the United States, although the
differences in the two populations are not as great as those
between Yakama and whites. Yakama had a high infant mortality rate throughout most of the twentieth century and continued to suffer high infant mortality into the 1960s.

Gender and blood quantum also were factors influencing
causes of death on the Yakama Reservation. Deaths of full-
bloods constituted 84 percent of all deaths between 1888 and
1964, and their numbers within the death population offer a
solid sample (figure 3.16). Most Indian people included in this
study were full-bloods. It is revealing to note that full–bloods
died less often of heart disease and cancer than did mixed-
bloods in relation to their percentage within the Yakama population. Full-bloods also died of automobile accidents at a
slightly higher percentage than their percentage within the
population. While 84 percent of the Yakama death population
from 1888 to 1964 was full-blood, a total of 86 percent of all
deaths resulting from automobile accidents was experienced by
full-bloods. More important, full-bloods died in large numbers
from influenza, accounting for 97 percent of all deaths resulting
from that disease. This is significant because the introduction of
new viruses seems to have affected full-bloods more than

mixed-bloods. The number of mixed-bloods within the death population is so small that it makes constructive comparisons difficult and, perhaps, unreliable. For this reason, a discussion of deaths in relationship to blood quantum is offered in an Appendix.

In comparison, the data relating to causes of death and gender is accurate and informative. Males and females died most often from tuberculosis, pneumonia, and heart disease. Females died more often of tuberculosis than did males, but males died more often than females of pneumonia—particularly male infants. The leading causes of death among females and males differ importantly after the first three causes of death mentioned above. Females died more often from cancer, with 71 percent of all cancer deaths experienced by women. They died primarily of uterine, stomach, breast, and cervical cancer (figure 4.6). Although these descriptions of cancer deaths are drawn from clinical explanations of death rather than medical explanations, they are revealing in terms of causes of death affecting different sexes. Females also died more often than males of meningitis and strokes. And childbirth was the ninth leading killer of women on the reservation (figure 3.11). Males died more often than females as a result of premature births, miscellaneous accidents, automobile accidents, and alcohol-related accidents and diseases. Gender roles and work habits probably account for some of these differences in number and causes of death.

The study ends in the year 1964, because Death Certificates were available in the National Archives, Pacific Northwest Region, only to this date. There is no question that a follow-up study using Death Certificates for the years after 1964 would be instructive to Yakama and to scholars, but such a study would require a researcher to examine every death recorded in Yakima County from 1965 to the present. It would require the researcher to be able to identify every member of the Yakama Nation who died in the county before the documents were coded. This would be a monumental task but one that would reveal many trends in Yakama health. In such a study, one might examine the importance the Hanford Nuclear Plant has had on the health of Yakama people due to the dumping of over 400 billion gallons of contaminated water into the soil on lands adjacent to the Columbia River and the release of radioactive gas into the air from the 1940s to the 1960s. Some people have suggested that the health of Yakama people has been placed at risk as a result of Hanford, and a death study of the people from 1964 to the 1990s would tell us much about this hypothesis. Clearly, there is more work to be done, but the present study will provide tribal people and scholars with a data base from which to investigate in the future.

During much of the twentieth century, the Yakama Reservation was a dangerous place to live, because no comparative data is available regarding death of Yakama Indians in urban areas or those off the reservation in rural areas, it is impossible to conclude that the Yakama Reservation was a more dangerous place to live than other places. Nevertheless, an analysis of the Death Certificates indicates that although the general Yakama population grew during the late nineteenth and early twentieth centuries—due to high birth rates, the migration of Indians onto the Yakama Reservation, and better public and medical health care—a large number of people died of diseases that were controlled in the general population of the United States but not on this Indian reservation. In addition, deaths by miscellaneous accidents and automobile accidents were also high on the Yakama Reservation (figure 3.2, 3.3, 4.4). Often crude death rates and infant mortality rates among Yakama were many times higher than those among other populations in the United States, and Yakama death statistics appear more like those of third world countries than a population within the borders of the United States. Statistics drawn from Yakama Death Certificates suggest that an argument could be made that this reservation fits soundly into the theory of internal colonialism, but this theory has not been explored in this work.[2]

Since 1964, the Indian Health Service and the Yakama Indian Health Center have made tremendous advances improving health conditions on the Yakama Reservation. Many changes actually began on 5 August 1954 with Public Law 83-568, the Transfer Act, which provided "that all functions, responsibilities, authorities, and duties . . . of hospitals and health facilities for Indians, and the conservation of Indian health . . . shall be administered by the Surgeon General and the United States Public Health Service."[3] As a result, since the 1960s, the Indian Health Service—a branch of the United States Public Health Service—has provided numerous programs designed to improve

Indian health through prevention, public health, rehabilitation, and curing.[4] On the Yakama Reservation, the Indian Health Service has offered programs designed to improve Indian health.[5] The Indian Health Service has built and renovated medical facilities, including a small but modern hospital at Toppenish, and improved sanitary and water systems. The Yakama Indian Health Center has also provided educational materials and programs regarding the HIV infection, infant car seats, safety belts, motorcycle helmets, water safety devices, agricultural equipment safety, pesticides, drug-alcohol abuse, and smoke-detection devices. The Indian Health Service and Yakama Indian Health Center have supported nutritional and dietary programs on the reservation stressing the importance of diet in one's health, particularly as a preventive measure against disease. In addition, the role of nurses and field educators on the Yakama Reservation has been expanded with positive results. In fact, crude death rates resulting from certain diseases have declined remarkably from 1964 to 1996.

Yakama people experienced two major dietary and nutritional transitions in the nineteenth and twentieth centuries. The first historical nutritional transition began in the nineteenth century with white contact and continued into the twentieth century. This was the era of white invasion, conquest, and resettlement of native lands, a time when non-Indians destroyed root and berry grounds through ranching and farming. During the nineteenth century, Yakama people began losing their lands and resources, the basis of their food supply. Moreover, Yakama people lost access to hunting grounds and fishing areas, lands that became part of the public domain, private property, or fell under the jurisdiction of state and/or federal officials who limited use of the land by Native Americans. In the twentieth century, the government of the United States destroyed fishing areas through dam projects. State officials arrested Indian hunters and fishers who practiced their ancient seasonal rounds in defiance of state laws but in accordance with federal treaty rights that secured for them their right to hunt and fish at all usual and accustomed areas. Their lives depended on the seasonal rounds, but state and federal governments ignored traditional customs and treaty rights, turning their backs on the ultimate consequences of such actions—the ill health of Yakama people.

In sum, Yakama people gradually lost their traditional food sources—foods high in vitamins, fiber, and carbohydrates, and low in saturated fats—during the late nineteenth and early twentieth centuries. During the course of the twentieth century, they relied more heavily on processed, refined foods which they purchased with cash or received as government commodities. They also ate beef and some pork which they raised on their own farms and ranches. This trend continued during the early twentieth century as Yakama families conducted limited farming, gardening, and stock raising for sale and for their own use. In addition, Yakama people—men, women, and children—worked as farm laborers. In the twentieth century, Yakama people worked as day laborers and farm laborers, earning cash which they used to purchase food.

Nutritional transitions accelerated with the twentieth century as Yakama hunting, fishing, and gathering complex gave way to one based on the consumption of processed foods. In the 1940s, several Yakama left the reservation to fight in World War II or work in defense plants. Some people continued to ranch, farm, fish, hunt, and gather, but wage earning took on a new meaning during and after World War II because of "modernization" and the destruction of root and berry grounds, the closure of hunting areas, and regulations placed on fishing. Much has been written on the destruction of the buffalo on the Great Plains and the collapse of the hunting complex among native peoples there. This is tantamount to what happened on the Columbia River Plateau, where the destruction of the hunting-fishing-gathering complex of Yakama Indians and their neighbors significantly changed the diet and way of life of Native Americans.[6]

After World War II, epidemiological and nutritional transitions changed rapidly for Yakama people, and this fact is reflected in major changes in causes of death among the native population on the reservation. The destruction of their traditional diet and greater use of processed foods led to a new era for Yakama people. After World War II, there was a "shift from a pattern of high prevalence of infectious diseases associated with malnutrition [tuberculosis, influenza, and gastrointestinal disorders], and with periodic famine and poor environmental sanitation, to a pattern of high prevalence of chronic and degenerative diseases." In addition, a major shift had occurred in the Yakama diet from traditional foods to processed foods, and this dietary change resulted in "a pattern of diet high in saturated fat, sugar, and refined foods and low in fiber" which is associated with man–made, degenerative diseases.[7]

Barry Popkin has argued that this is a part of a human pattern of nutritional transitions, when people eat a "diet high in total fat, cholesterol, sugar, and other refined carbohydrates and low in polyunsaturated fatty acids and fiber, often accompanied by increasingly sedentary life."[8] Nutritional transitions coincided with epidemiological transitions during World War II, as deaths resulting from tuberculosis and gastrointestinal disorders gave way as major causes of death to heart disease and cancer. In addition, with "modernization" and a cash economy came increased numbers of accidental, automobile deaths, which had been an important cause of death throughout the twentieth century but took on even greater meaning after World War II. What was most striking were new causes of death that took center stage by the 1980s and 1990s. Although heart disease, pneumonia, and accidental deaths continued to be important causes of death between 1964 and 1994, suicides and murders grew to epidemic proportions.

The best information on Yakama Indian health in recent years is contained in an informative document entitled "1991 Mortality Report" compiled by John Moran, Sharon John, Jim Horst, Evelyn Broncheau, Karen Schmidt, Jim Sutherland, Linda Kofford, Corky Covington, and Pam Garza. Drawing on Death Certificates, obituaries, tribal enrollment information, and information "obtained through family members and other informal sources," the staff of the Yakama Indian Health Center offered the following data regarding morbidity and mortality from 1987 to 1991.[9] Overall, health on the Yakama Indian Reservation has improved dramatically since the 1950s, and there have been some shifts and consistencies in the causes of death. Major causes of death recorded in Death Certificates before World War II during the ages of Pestilence and Receding Pandemics were tuberculosis, influenza, gastrointestinal disorders, miscellaneous accidents, automobile accidents, premature births, and pneumonia. Since the 1950s, tuberculosis, gastrointestinal disorders, influenza, and premature births have nearly disappeared as causes of death, while pneumonia and accidents of all kinds continue to be major causes of death (figure 4.4).

During the era from 1964 to 1991, the Yakama Indian population has continued to grow, attaining a current total of approximately 14,700 people. Below are a few comparisons of causes of death and crude death rates for Yakama and American Indians-Alaskan Natives within the service area of the Indian Health Service. In 1990, the crude death rate per 100,000 in the Yakama population resulting from heart disease was 75 (N = 15), while it was 112 (average, 1986-88) for Native Americans. Thus, compared to other native people, Yakama had a death rate resulting from heart disease well below the national average for native people.[10] This pattern was also true in 1990 for crude death rates per 100,000 in the Yakama population for strokes and cancer. Yakama experienced a crude death rate from strokes of 20, while other Native Americans had a crude death rate of 22. The Yakama had a crude death rate of 34 resulting from cancer, while other native peoples had a death rate of 66. However, Yakama crude death rates for accidental deaths, homicides, suicides, and pneumonia were higher in 1990 than those for other Native Americans.[11]

The following data offers comparisons of age-adjusted mortality rates per 100,000 in the population between the Yakama in 1991, Native Americans within the service area of the Indian Health Service in 1988, and the general population of the United States in 1989, as provided by the Yakama Indian Health Center. All comparisons are for these three different years. The age adjusted-mortality rate resulting from all forms of accidental death (miscellaneous and automobile) among the Yakama was 92 (N = 13), while it was 81 among other native populations and 34 within the general population of the United States. Although the number of cases within the Yakama population is low in comparison to other populations, the mortality rate is higher. Clearly, deaths resulting from miscellaneous and automobile accidents continued to be high among Yakama people, just as they had been since the 1930s. However, because of the decline of other causes of death, most notably tuberculosis, influenza, and premature births, deaths caused by accidents have taken on new significance in the epidemiological transition of Yakama people. Like accidental deaths, pneumonia continued to affect the Yakama population from the 1960s to the 1990s. In 1991, the age-adjusted mortality rate among Yakama people due to accidental deaths was 75 (N = 5), while it was 19 among other Native Americans and 13 within the general population of the United States. Therefore, in spite of advances in health education programs, medical care, and medicine, Yakama people continued to die at a higher rate than other populations as a result of accidental deaths and pneumonia.[12]

One major change in terms of causes of death marked the era from 1964 to 1991. From 1888 to 1964, homicide was not a major cause of death. Of the 23 Yakama people (N = 12 females, 11 males) who died as a result of murder during the seventy-six-year period, murders included 5 teenagers, 3 were in their twenties, 5 in their thirties, 2 in their forties, and 4 in their fifties. Historically, 6 Yakama were murdered during the 1920s, 7 in the 1930s, 5 in the 1940s, and 5 in the 1950s. Between 1960 and 1964, there were no Yakama reported in Death Certificates to have died as a result of homicide. However, in 1991, the age adjusted mortality rate resulting from homicide was 26 (N = 5), while it was 14 among other Native Americans and 9 in the general population of the United States. Thus, in 1991 alone, Yakama experienced as many deaths as they had during the 1940s and 1950s. The staff of the Yakama Indian Health Center was alarmed at the number of homicides, particularly when they learned that homicides were occurring in the age group between 15 and 34 years of age. This was also the case for suicides among Yakama people.[13]

During the era from 1888 to 1964, suicide was not a major cause of death among Yakama people. During the seventy-six-year period, a total of 19 Yakama (N = 11 males, 8 females) took their own lives. Of those Yakama that died as a result of suicide, 2 were teenagers, 8 were in their twenties, 5 were in their thirties, 2 were in their forties, and 1 each were in their fifties and sixties. During this era, 1 person committed suicide in the 1910s, 5 in the 1920s, 4 in the 1930s, 1 in the 1940s, 7 in the 1950s, and 1 between 1960 and 1964. Thus, historically, suicide was not a great killer of Yakama people, but in the 1990s, this cause of death reached epidemic proportions. The medical staff of the Yakama Indian Health Center reported that in 1991, suicide reached an alarming rate. The age-adjusted mortality rate resulting from suicide per 100,000 in the population was 40 (N = 6) among Yakama, 19 among other native peoples, and 13 within the general population of the United States. Researchers at the Yakama Indian Health Center reported that "there is excessive mortality from unintentional injury as well as from homicide and suicide."[14]

In 1991, the researchers contend that "the one-year cancer death rate is well below half of the United States all races rate."[15] Between the era from 1888 to 1964, cancer was a leading cause of death on the Yakama Reservation, but its significance as a cause of death climbed between 1950 and 1964 (N = 33/40 percent). In 1991, the age-adjusted mortality rate resulting from cancer among Yakama was 52 (N = 5), while it was 91 (in 1988) among Native Americans and 134 (in 1989) within the general population of the United States. Thus, as in past decades, although cancer was an important cause of death and although cancer rose in importance as a cause of death among Yakama people, it was not as acute among the Yakama population as it was among other populations. This trend has continued throughout most of the twentieth century. In addition to cancer-related deaths, there were 3 deaths resulting from diabetes. The number of deaths may not appear large, but diabetes has grown in importance as a cause of death. As Eugene S. Hunn has pointed out, "biological assaults on Plateau Indian populations did not cease with the waning of brutal epidemics of smallpox, measles, and assorted scourges." He maintains that in recent years "a new and more insidious biological hazard has begun," and "this modern epidemic is diabetes."[16] Hunn argues that diabetes "may not kill outright, but is closely correlated with an increased incidence of heart disease, high blood pressure associated with obesity, and gall bladder disease."[17]

Diabetes has become a significant cause of death among many Native American populations in the late twentieth century, including Yakama. The rise of diabetes may be the result of nutritional transitions and genetic makeup of native peoples. The consumption of "processed foods that are high in short-chain carbohydrates and animal fats but low in long-chain carbohydrates and fiber" may be a cause of the rise in diabetes on the Yakama Reservation.[18] Since food is considered sacred by Yakama people, families emphasize that it should not be wasted but totally consumed. Indeed, food was to be shared by all in feasting, an act that was also considered sacred. Since World War II, Yakama people have consumed more and more processed foods, sometimes eating in excess of their needs. This, as well as a genetic predisposition to the disease, may have contributed to the rise in diabetes. Geneticist James Neel has suggested that hunting and gathering cultures—like Yakama—may have a genetic makeup which includes a "diabetes gene."[19] Hunn theorizes that Yakama and other native peoples may have social and biological mechanisms at work that contribute to the rise in deaths related to diabetes.[20] In 1991, the age adjusted mortality rate resulting from diabetes per 100,000 in the Yakama population was 35 (N=3), while it was 26 (in 1988) among other Native Americans and 11 (in 1989) within the general population of the United States. Thus, although the total number of deaths was small, the death rate was higher than for other native peoples and other Americans within the United States.[21]

In addition, as Gregory R. Campbell indicates, "Type II diabetes mellitus is a new disease among Native American people." He maintains that, prior to 1940, few cases of diabetes were recorded for American Indians, and this is certainly true on the Yakama Reservation where diabetes was not recorded once as a cause of death in the Death Certificates before 1940. Campbell argues that, since World War II, adult onset diabetes "has become a major epidemic" and "currently [1989] the seventh leading cause of death among Native Americans, exceeding 2.8 times the United States all races age–adjusted mortality rate." The disease is also debilitating, causing blindness, cataracts, amputations, renal disease, and heart problems.[22] James W. Justice has pointed out that diabetes began within Native American populations as traditional food sources became scarce and refined foods became more available.[23] He is correct, and this is exactly what occurred on the Yakama Reservation during the 1940s.

The second phase of diabetes among the Native American population emerged when foods became increasingly available, particularly foods high in fats and carbohydrates. Adults have a tendency to become obese and elementary children become overweight with high blood sugar. Soon, Justice argues, young women who were obese began having children, and their condition produced the fourth and fifth phases of diabetes in a population in which increased obesity and diabetes contribute to more "uterine cancer, en–stage renal diseases, amputations, and hypertension."[24] Justice has studied diabetes on the Warm

Springs Reservation of central Oregon, arguing that this population is in phase three of the disease. This is also the case for Yakama people and other Native American nations in the Northwest. Diabetes—a disease resulting, in part, from ample food supplies, cash to purchase refined foods high in calories, and less exercise—will continue to be present on Northwestern reservations unless sufficient resources are committed to the problem. The return to a traditional diet is one key to facing diabetes, but it is a difficult task indeed due to the destruction of native roots, berries, game, and fish. Diabetes is a result of epidemiological and nutritional transitions that have been detrimental to Yakama people.

In addition to diabetes, researchers of the Yakama Indian Health Center considered other important aspects of mortality on the reservation in 1991. They maintain that deaths resulting from cardiovascular diseases among all Yakama are about equal to those in the general population of the United States. They also argue, as pointed out above, that the death rate from cancer is less than one-half that of the general population of the United States. All of these aspects of Yakama mortality mirror statistics found historically in the Yakama population during the early twentieth century, although rates of death vary according to the time period within the era from 1888 to 1964.[25] And while cancer became an increasingly important cause of death among Yakama during the last fourteen years covered by this study, it was not as important as it was within the general population of the United States. However, crude death rates from all forms of accidental death among Yakama of all ages was high throughout the course of the twentieth century and continue to be a major cause of death within the Yakama population today.

The mortality report of the Yakama Indian Health Center revealed that there was considerable mortality in the age group between 15 and 34. Between 1987 and 1991, the death rate in this age group was "nearly three times the U. S. all races mortality."[26] The leading killers of this age group during this five year period were accidents of all kinds (N = 36/55 percent) and homicide–suicide (N = 20/31 percent). Together, these causes of death accounted for 86 percent of all deaths experienced by Yakama between the ages of 15 and 34. Throughout the period from 1888 to 1964, this age group was particularly vulnerable to high rates of mortality, but it was primarily tuberculosis that preyed on this age group—principally from 1924 to 1944. In addition, during the course of the twentieth century, this age group also suffered numerous deaths due to miscellaneous accidents and automobile accidents. But Yakama people between the ages of 15 and 34 did not suffer many deaths each year from homicides and suicides, not in the pre-World War II period and not in the postwar-period to 1964. The rising number of deaths in this age group resulting from suicides and murders is a new and dangerous trend, one that is not reflected in the historical data from past Death Certificates.

Researchers at the Yakama Indian Health Center concluded their work on mortality by stating that the most significant finding in their study of the five-year period from 1987 to 1991 was "the disturbing high death rate among young people, ages 15 to 34." Of the 65 deaths experienced by this age group, "More than half [of] these deaths were accidental, a third were due to either homicide or suicide." The researchers asserted that drug and alcohol use "were felt to be factor[s] in a majority of these deaths."[27] In addition to these deaths, another 5 people died as a result of alcohol. The medical staff of the Yakama Indian Health Center have tried to devise "strategies to curb driving while intoxicated."[28] Deaths resulting from alcohol and drug use have grown considerably among Yakama people since the 1960s. In the early twentieth century, deaths resulting from drug and alcohol use were not great (N=51 from 1888-1964), but clearly, this cause of death has become a leading killer among the people.

Epidemiological transitions are well marked in the nineteenth and twentieth centuries among Yakama Indians. In the late nineteenth and early twentieth centuries, white resettlement of Indian lands and government Indian policies destroyed root, berry, fishing, and hunting grounds. Traditional food resources diminished with time as the government confined Indians more and more to their reservation. Ranching, farming, canal construction, road building, dam projects, etc. all contributed to the decline of natural food sources for Yakama people. All of these aspects of Western American history have been heralded in the past as positive elements of westward expansion and the winning of the west. But all of these products of "civilization" and "progress" have been detrimental to Native

Americans, including members of the Confederated Tribes of the Yakama Nation.

The epidemiological and nutritional history of the Yakama has been adversely affected by the introduction of contagious diseases, creation of the reservation, consolidation of several tribes and bands onto a single land base, the absence of public and medical health, and the destruction of traditional foods by white farmers, ranchers, timber companies, etc. Government policies and white resettlement of the Columbia Plateau ended seasonal rounds. Indian policies, diseases, and Christian missionaries diminished the importance of midwives and medicine people. White rule of Yakama people by agents of the United States government led to anomie that negatively influenced the mental, physical, and spiritual health of native people, making the Yakama more susceptible to tuberculosis, pneumonia, heart disease, and gastrointestinal disorders. A vicious cycle emerged on the Yakama Reservation as societal depression increased with the number of deaths, particularly those of infants and children under six years of age. The greater the anomie, the more susceptible the people were to disease and death—and later alcohol, suicide, and murder. Still, in spite of high death rates and infant mortality rates, the Yakama population persevered and recovered, growing steadily after the 1930s.

Although the total number of deaths among Yakama each year has declined in recent years, the people continue to live at risk. Economic and health conditions have generally improved on the Yakama Reservation since the 1950s, but the people spent the first half of the twentieth century living on a reservation that was unhealthy and dangerous, a place where large numbers of people died—especially infants and children under six years of age. In spite of conditions on the reservation, many Yakama survived and strengthened the population so that the Yakama Nation exists to this day. But the health problems of the past have not been forgotten by the people, and this work provides a voice for the Yakama dead. Every family recalls the death of loved ones as a result of tuberculosis, pneumonia, accidents, and a host of other causes. Elders remember the epidemics of the twentieth century. They remember diseases that preyed on their families and friends, wrenching the lives out of infants and children. They understand all too well what is meant by high death rates, high fetal death rates, and high infant mortality rates. Better than anyone else, they know that death stalked the Yakama during the late nineteenth and early twentieth centuries.

Notes

1. Omran, "Epidemiologic Transition in the United States," 16–17.

2. John R. Weeks to Clifford E. Trafzer, 15 June 1994, author's collection.

3. Indian Health Service, "Trends in Indian Health," 1.

4. Ibid.

5. Ibid.

6. Omran, "Epidemiologic Transition in the United States," 16–18; Popkin, "Nutritional Patterns and Transitions," 138–45; Hunn, *Nch'i-Wana*, 282–94.

7. Popkin, "Nutritional Patterns and Transitions," 138.

8. Ibid., 139.

9. John Moran, et al., "Yakima Indian Health Center 1991 Mortality Report," Public Health Service, Indian Health Service, Yakama Service Area, 401 Buster Road, Toppenish, Wash., 1991, p. 1 (hereafter cited as Moran, "1991 Mortality Report").

10. Ibid., 3.

11. Ibid.

12. Ibid., 6.

13. Ibid.

14. Ibid., 7.

15. Ibid.

16. Hunn, *Nch'i-Wana*, 282.

17. Ibid., 283.

18. Ibid.

19. James V. Neel, "Diabetes Mellitus: A 'Thrifty' Genotype Rendered Detrimental by 'Progress,' "*American Journal of Human Genetics* 14 (1962): 353–62.

20. Hunn, *Nch'i-Wana*, 284.

21. Moran, "1991 Mortality Report," 6; for an excellent discussion of the importance of diabetes on another Northwestern Indian reservation, see James W. Justice, "Twenty Years of Diabetes on the Warm Springs Indian Reservation, Oregon," *American Indian Culture and Research Journal* 13 (1989): 49–81.

22. Gregory R. Campbell, "The Changing Dimensions of Native American Health: A Critical Understanding of Contemporary Native American Health Issues," *American Indian Culture and Research Journal* 13 (1989): 9.

23. Justice, "Twenty Years of Diabetes on the Warm Springs Reservation, Oregon," 72.

24. Ibid., 73.

25. Moran, "1991 Mortality Report," 6, 10, 11.

26. Ibid., 10.

27. Ibid., 12.

28. Ibid.

APPENDIX

Impact of Blood Quantum on Yakama Deaths

Many of the Death Certificates included information regarding a person's blood quantum, place of death, tribal affiliation, and enrollment status. The most important of these variables was blood quantum, since scholars generally hold that full-bloods died more frequently from diseases introduced by non-Indians than people of mixed-Indian and white blood. One scholar has asserted that "many mixed-bloods [Yakama] were granted fee patents to their lands and considered citizens and therefore outside the scope of federal reservation jurisdiction" and that the data from the Death Certificates used in this study do not reflect deaths of mixed-blood Yakama.[1] It is true that the present study focuses on the reservation, but it is not true that the Plateau Indians who filed for land under the Indian Homestead Act were mixed-bloods. Wenatchi, Palouse, Sincayuse, Walula, Wanapum, and other Indians from the mid-Columbia River region filed homesteads, but most of these families were not Yakama, although many of them were supposed to have removed to the Yakama Reservation, and some did during the course of the twentieth century. Thus, some of the Indians who filed homesteads lost their lands and moved to the reservation. Others, like the extended family of Mary Jim, were forced onto the Yakama Reservation by federal officials who condemned her land for reclamation projects in the 1960s. Few—if any—of these families were of mixed Indian-white blood. They were primarily full-bloods, and most were not Yakama, since many Yakama chose to remain on the reservation to live with families and friends who were of the same tribal affiliation as themselves. To track each of these families to acquire their Death Certificates would be an overwhelming task, and it would have little influence on this data dealing with blood quantum and death among the Yakama population on the reservation.

It is tempting to make the argument that Yakama full-bloods on the reservation died more often of disease than people of mixed-blood. According to the data, full-bloods on the Yakama Indian Reservation died more often than mixed-bloods of each of the ten leading causes of death: tuberculosis, pneumonia, heart diseases, miscellaneous accidents, gastrointestinal disorders, automobile accidents, influenza, cancer, premature birth, and senility. Since most of the Indians living on the Yakama Reservation were enrolled as full-bloods, more full-bloods died of all causes of death. The major flaw in pointing out the strong relationship between full-bloods and death by all causes is that full-bloods comprised over 80 percent of the death population whose blood quantum was known. However, of the 3,899 cases found in the Death Certificates, the blood quantum of only 2,640 is known. Of these, 2,213 (84 percent) were full-bloods, 263 (10 percent) were of half-blood or more but less than full, and 164 (6 percent) were one quarter-bloods. Although deaths by smallpox, childbirth, and whooping cough were not among the ten most frequent causes of death, it is important to recognize that nearly all the deaths by these causes were suffered by full-bloods. Between 1888 and 1964, 3 (100 percent) full-bloods died of smallpox, 15 (83 percent) died in childbirth, and 16 (94 percent) died of whooping cough.

The leading cause of death among Yakama people between 1888 and 1964 was tuberculosis. A total of 394 (80 percent) full-bloods died and 57 (12 percent) people of half or more Yakama bloods succumbed to the disease. By comparison, 41 (8 percent) quarter-bloods died of tuberculosis. Full-bloods were susceptible to tubercle bacteria just as they were to those causing pneumonia, the second leading cause of death on the Yakama Reservation. Of the 366 people who died of pneumonia, 309 (84 percent) were full-bloods, 43 (12 percent) were half or more but less than full, and 14 (4 percent) were quarter-bloods. Thus, the percentage of death among full-bloods who died of tuberculosis and pneumonia is about the same as that of their percentage in the Yakama population. Full-bloods also died more often of heart disease, although the percentage of their deaths is less than their percentage within the Yakama population where blood quantum was known. Of the 155 Yakama people who died of heart diseases, 108 (70 percent) were full-bloods, 34 (22 percent) were half or more but less than full, and 13 (8 percent) were quarter-bloods. The fact that the percentage of full-bloods who died of heart disease was lower than their percent within the Yakama death population may have been linked to diet.

Although this remains speculative, it might have been the case that full-bloods on the whole were more traditional in their diets than mixed-bloods, preferring to hunt, fish, and gather rather than eating processed foods or foods high in fat, like beef and pork. The Death Certificates are mute on these points, but the diet of full-bloods and their use of little tobacco may offer clues to lower numbers of deaths resulting from heart disease. The dietary habits of full-bloods and mixed-bloods in the historical context are difficult to determine, but this is certainly a possibility worth consideration, particularly because most full-bloods practiced the Washat, which emphasized the consumption of salmon, roots, and berries.

Miscellaneous accidents and gastrointestinal disorders accounted for the fourth and fifth leading causes of death in the Yakama population, and full-bloods experienced the majority of deaths resulting from these causes. However, like heart diseases, the percentage of those full-bloods who died from these two causes is less than the percentage of full-bloods within the Yakama population. This was also the case for cancer and premature births, the eighth and ninth leading causes of death on the Yakama Reservation. A total of 84 people died by accidents, 62 (74 percent) of whom were full-bloods, 11 (13 percent) were half or more but less than full, and 11 (13 percent) were quarter-bloods.

Again, it may be speculated that full-bloods died less often of accidental deaths because they pursued a more traditional life style. They likely earned their living through hunting, fishing, and gathering, rather than by wage earning. Taking and consuming foods in the traditional manner was more than an economic issue among Yakama people and other Indians of the Columbia Plateau. It was a religious act, recreating the relationship of humans with the creative powers of plants and animals in accordance with ancient stories and tribal traditions.

It may be that full-bloods felt a greater relationship to this way of life than mixed-bloods, but the evidence through an examination of the Death Certificates neither confirms nor denies this theory. Also related to food, water, and the relationship of humans to the environment are gastrointestinal disorders. A total of 67 Yakama Indians died of gastrointestinal disorders, 49 (73 percent) of whom were full-bloods, 14 (21 percent) were half or more but less than full, and 4 (6 percent) were one quarter-bloods.

A similar situation is found for those Yakama that died of cancer and premature births. Of the 38 people who died of cancer, 22 (58 percent) were full-bloods, 8 (21 percent) were half or more but less than full, and 8 (21 percent) were quarter-bloods. The fact that full-bloods comprised 84 percent of the Yakama death population but suffered only 58 percent of the deaths resulting from cancer may indicate that the diets of full-bloods might account in part for fewer deaths resulting from various types of cancer. And of the 34 people who died as a result of premature birth and whose blood quantum was known, 25 (74 percent) were full-bloods, 5 (15 percent) were half or more but less than full, and 4 (11 percent) were quarter-bloods. In the case of deaths by miscellaneous accidents, gastrointestinal disorders, cancer, and premature births, the percentage of deaths among full-bloods was less than their percentage in the population. Conversely, for those Yakama whose blood quantum was less than that of the full-bloods, their percentage of deaths by these various causes was higher than their percentage within the Yakama death population.

Full-bloods constituted 84 percent of the Yakama death population, and they died of automobile accidents in about equal proportion to their percentage within the population. Death by automobile accidents was the sixth most frequent cause of death on the Yakama Reservation. Of the 42 people who died from automobile accidents, 36 (86 percent) were full-bloods, 4 (10 percent) were half or more but less than full, and 2 (4 percent) were quarter-bloods. Thus, people died in roughly equal proportion to their percentage within the population. However, in the case of influenza and senility, the percentage of deaths among full-bloods from these two causes was higher than their percentage within the Yakama population. Influenza was the seventh leading cause of death, and senility was the tenth most frequent cause of death. Of the 93 people who died of influenza, 90 (97 percent) were full-bloods, 1 (1 percent) was half or more but less than full, and 2 (2 percent) were one quarter-bloods. This is an incredible percentage of deaths from influenza among full-bloods and most likely was the result of biological factors. Influenza viruses definitely affected far more full-bloods than mixed-bloods, but influenza was a major killer only for those years from 1900 until the 1930s, a time when most of the population was composed of full-bloods. In the case of senility, of the 54 people who died of this cause, 53 (98 percent) were full-bloods, 0 were half or more but less than full, and 1 (2 percent) person was of one-quarter Indian blood. Perhaps full-bloods lived longer and died of old age, a cause of death designated as senility in the early twentieth century.

Clearly, the blood quantum of an individual had some affect on the cause of death, but it is not apparent from the data that full-bloods were more likely to die of most diseases, except influenza, than mixed-bloods. In the cases of influenza and senility, a larger percentage of full-bloods died than their percentage within the Yakama population. However, in every other case—except for automobile accidents—the percentage of deaths of full-bloods by the various other causes of death in the top ten category was equal to or less than the percentage of full-bloods within the Yakama population.

Appendix Note

1.   Reader's Report, "Death Stalks the Yakama," 3 November 1993.

Figure 1.1. Number of death certificates, 1888-1964

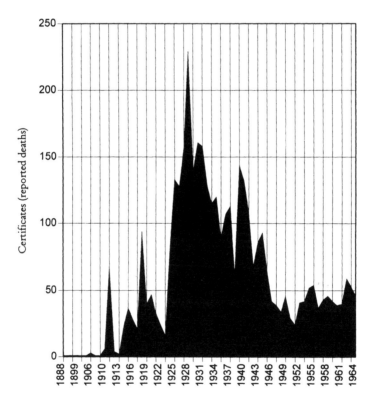

Figure 1.2. **Leading causes of Yakama death, 1888-1964**

Cause	Number of Deaths	Percent
Tuberculosis	619	28.0%
Pneumonia	566	25.6%
Heart Diseases	325	14.7%
Misc. Accidents	145	6.6%
Gastrointestinal	124	5.6%
Automobile accidents	122	5.5%
Influenza	104	4.7%
Cancer	82	3.7%
Premature birth	64	2.9%
Senility	57	2.6%
Total	2208	99.9%

Figure 1.3. **Leading causes of Yakama death by age group**

Age	Tuberculosis	Pneumonia	Heart Disease	Misc. Accidents	Gastro-intestinal
< 5	56	344	20	17	105
5-9	35	18	3	2	3
10-14	48	3	5	4	0
15-19	112	5	0	9	1
20-24	88	10	4	18	0
25-29	65	12	5	17	1
30-34	28	2	2	9	3
35-39	36	6	13	4	0
40-44	18	17	13	11	1
45-49	24	12	18	14	0
50-54	21	13	16	8	0
55-59	26	23	26	7	1
60-64	15	10	31	1	1
65-69	12	19	35	4	1
70-74	11	19	32	7	1
75-79	13	18	34	5	3
> 80	7	32	65	5	3
Total	615	563	322	142	124

Figure 1.4. **Yakama tuberculosis deaths by age group and gender**

Age	Female	Row Percentage	Male	Row Percentage	Total
< 5	35	63%	21	37%	56
5-9	18	51%	17	49%	35
10-14	29	58%	17	42%	48
15-19	45	40%	67	60%	112
20-24	40	45%	48	55%	88
25-29	35	54%	30	46%	65
30-34	17	61%	11	39%	28
35-39	25	69%	11	31%	36
40-44	10	55%	8	45%	18
45-49	14	61%	9	39%	23
50-54	14	67%	7	33%	21
55-59	13	50%	13	50%	26
60-64	7	47%	8	53%	15
65-69	7	58%	5	42%	12
70-74	6	55%	5	45%	11
75-79	8	61%	5	39%	13
> 80	4	57%	3	43%	7
Total	327		287		614

Figure 1.5. **Yakama pneumonia deaths by age group and gender**

Age	Female	Row Percentage	Male	Row Percentage	Total
< 5	130	38%	214	62%	344
5-9	10	56%	8	44%	18
10-14	2	67%	1	33%	3
15-19	5	100%	0	0%	5
20-24	1	10%	9	90%	10
25-29	8	67%	4	33%	12
30-34	2	100%	0	0%	2
35-39	6	100%	0	0%	6
40-44	7	44%	9	56%	16
45-49	8	67%	4	33%	12
50-54	2	15%	11	85%	13
55-59	11	48%	12	52%	23
60-64	1	10%	9	90%	10
65-69	10	53%	9	47%	19
70-74	7	37%	12	63%	19
75-79	10	11%	84	89%	94
> 80	19	59%	13	41%	32
Total	239		399		638

Figure 1.6. Infant mortality rates, Yakama, non-whites,
and State of Washington, 1914-1964

Year	Yakama	Births/ Death <1	Whites	Non-Whites	State of Washington
1914	500	2/1	NA	NA	NA
1919	375	8/3	83	131	63
1921	77	13/1	73	109	55
1923	429	7/3	74	117	57
1926	444	36/16	70	112	56
1927	684	19/13	61	100	50
1928	474	57/27	64	106	48
1929	384	73/28	63	102	49
1930	564	55/31	60	100	49
1931	373	83/31	57	93	48
1932	316	95/30	53	86	45
1933	209	91/19	53	91	39
1934	193	86/16	55	94	43
1935	270	89/24	52	83	45
1936	127	63/8	53	88	45
1937	167	60/10	50	83	45
1938	173	81/14	47	79	40
1939	389	72/28	44	74	39
1940	342	79/27	43	74	35
1941	276	87/24	41	75	34
1942	130	92/12	37	65	33
1943	101	119/12	38	63	35
1944	311	103/32	37	60	34
1945	103	107/11	36	57	35
1946	100	80/8	32	50	33
1947	68	88/6	30	49	28
1948	19	106/2	30	47	28
1949	117	103/12	29	47	27
1950	111	72/8	27	45	27
1951	32	62/2	26	45	24
1952	78	128/10	26	47	25
1953	104	96/10	25	47	25
1954	104	135/14	24	43	24
1955	133	120/16	24	43	23
1956	70	129/9	23	42	23
1957	85	130/11	23	44	23
1958	79	151/12	24	46	25
1959	31	162/5	23	44	23
1960	29	205/6	23	43	23
1961	40	174/7	22	41	22
1962	91	186/17	22	41	21
1963	76	144/11	22	42	22
1964	26	230/6	22	41	

Figure 1.7. **Yakama population growth, 1885-1980**

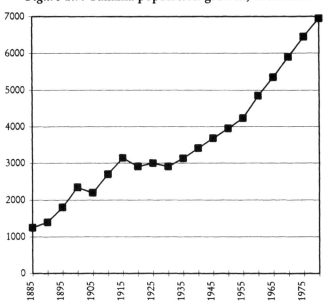

Note: Population totals for 1935, 1940, 1945, 1950, and 1955 are esti mates based on the assumption of linear population growth between the years 1932 and 1960

Figure 1.8. Yakama birth rates, 1915-1964

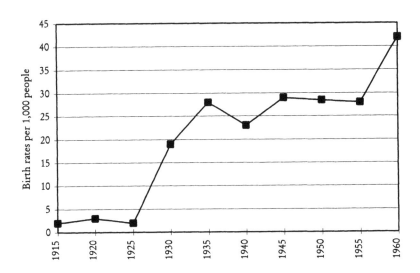

Figure 1.9. Yakama birth rates, 1915-1964

Year	Births	Population	Birth Rate (per 1,000)
1915	5	3,146	2
1920	9	2,910	3
1925	6	3,001	2
1930	55	2,908	19
1935	89	3,136	28
1940	79	3,411	23
1945	107	3,686	29
1955	120	4,236	28
1960	205	4,844	42
1964	230	5,508	42

Figure 1.10. Number of Yakama death certificates per year, 1888-1964

Year	Number	Year	Number	Year	Number	Year	Number
1888	1	1917	21	1933	115	1949	46
1890	1	1918	94	1934	120	1950	29
1895	1	1919	40	1935	89	1951	24
1899	1	1920	47	1936	107	1952	41
1900	1	1921	33	1937	113	1953	42
1901	1	1922	24	1938	61	1954	52
1906	3	1923	16	1939	144	1955	54
1908	1	1924	80	1940	132	1956	37
1909	1	1925	133	1941	108	1957	43
1910	6	1926	128	1942	68	1958	48
1911	68	1927	157	1943	86	1959	42
1912	4	1928	229	1944	93	1960	39
1913	2	1929	139	1945	65	1961	40
1914	23	1930	161	1946	42	1962	59
1915	37	1931	158	1947	39	1963	53
1916	28	1932	129	1948	34	1964	46

Figure 3.1. Yakama Miscellaneous Deaths by Age Group and Gender

Age	Female	Row Percentage	Male	Row Percentage	Total
< 5	7	41%	10	59%	17
5-9	2	100%	0	0%	2
10-14	1	25%	3	75%	4
15-19	2	22%	7	88%%	9
20-24	1	5%	17	95%	18
25-29	3	18%	14	82%	17
30-34	0	0%	9	100%	9
35-39	1	25%	3	75%	4
40-44	0	0%	11	100%	11
45-49	1	7%	13	93%	14
50-54	3	37%	5	63%	8
55-59	0	0%	7	100%	7
60-64	0	0%	1	100%	1
65-69	0	0%	4	100%	4
70-74	3	43%	4	57%	7
75-79	2	40%	3	60%	5
> 80	4	80%	1	20%	5
Total	30		112		142

*Figure 3.2.*Moving averages for miscellaneous accidents

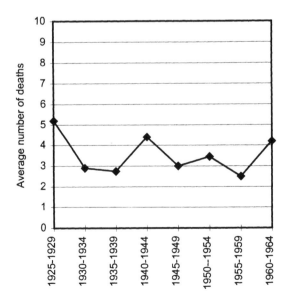

Figure 3.3. Moving averages for automobile accidents

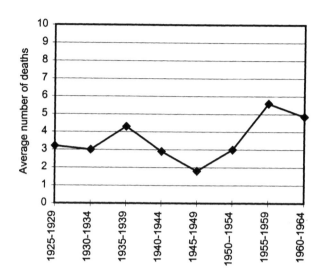

Figure 3.4. Moving averages for pneumonia

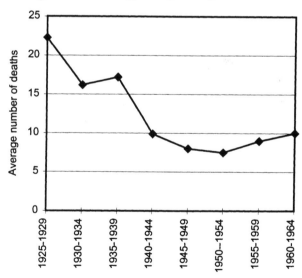

Figure 3.5. Yakama Birth Rates, 1915-1964

Year	Yakama	White US	Non-White US
1926	194	35	73
1927	105	35	75
1928	70	35	82
1929	27	34	80
1930	36	34	80
1931	60	33	74
1932	42	33	74
1936	143	30	67
1937	117	29	63
1938	25	28	61
1939	42	28	59
1940	63	28	57
1941	34	27	54
1942	54	26	49
1943	25	24	46
1944	29	25	45
1945	37	21	42
1946	25	20	41
1947	11	19	37
1948	19	18	37
1949	29	18	35
1953	21	16	30
1954	7	16	29
1955	8	15	28
1956	16	15	27
1957	15	15	27
1958	13	15	28
1960	24	14	27
1961	11	14	27
1962	22	14	27
1963	21	14	27
1964	13	14	28

Figure 3.6. Leading causes of death by gender for Yakama Children under one year of age

Cause	Males	Females	Total
Pneumonia	141 (66%)	74 (34%)	215 (29%)
Gastrointestinal	29 (44%)	37 (56%)	66 (9%)
Prematurity	8 (44%)	10 (56%)	18
Stillborn	9 (56%)	6 (44%)	15
Tuberculosis	9 (75%)	3 (25%)	12
Total	239	165	404

Figure 3.7. Leading causes of death by gender
for Yakama Children one year of age

Cause	Males	Females	Total
Pneumonia	37 (60%)	25 (40%)	62 (26%)
Gastrointestinal	16 (59%)	11 (41%)	27 (12%)
Tuberculosis	6 (40%)	9 (60%)	15 (6%)
Misc. Accidents	6 (75%)	2 (25%)	8 (3%)
Whooping Cough	4 (57%)	3 (43%)	7 (3%)
Total	69	50	119 (51%)

Figure 3.8. Leading causes of death by gender
for Yakama Children one year of age

Cause	Males	Females	Total
Pneumonia	37 (53%)	33 (47%)	70 (25%)
Tuberculosis	13 (39%)	20 (61%)	33 (12%)
Gastrointestinal	10 (67%)	5 (33%)	15 (5%)
Meningitis	9 (69%)	4 (31%)	13 (5%)
Misc. Accidents	4 (44%)	5 (56%)	9 (3%)
Total	73	67	140 (51%)

Figure 3.9. Number of Yakama deaths by age group, 1888-1964

Age	Number of Deaths	Percent
0 through 4	1,213	31
5 through 9	144	4
10 through 14	113	3
15 through 19	208	5
20 through 24	218	6
25 through 29	173	5
30 through 34	146	4
35 through 39	119	3
40 through 44	125	3
45 through 49	132	3
50 through 54	133	3
55 through 59	164	4
60 through 64	141	4
65 through 69	172	4
70 through 74	177	5
75 through 79	171	4
over 80	284	7
Total	3,833	67

Figure 3.10. Yakama premature births and still births
fetal death rate per 1,000 live births, selected years

Year	Births	Premature & Still Births	Rate per 1,000 live births
1912	na	1	na
1918	7	1	143
1926	36	7	194
1927	19	2	105
1928	57	4	70
1929	73	2	27
1930	55	2	36
1931	83	5	60
1932	95	4	42
1936	63	9	143
1937	60	7	117
1938	81	2	25
1939	72	3	42
1940	79	5	63
1941	87	3	34
1942	92	5	54
1943	119	3	25
1944	103	3	29
1945	107	4	37
1946	80	2	25
1947	88	1	11
1948	106	2	19
1949	103	3	29
1953	96	2	21
1954	135	1	7
1955	129	1	8
1956	129	2	16
1957	130	2	15
1958	151	2	13
1960	205	5	24
1961	174	2	11
1962	186	4	22
1963	144	3	21
1964	230	3	13

Figure 3.11. Leading Causes of death for females and males
in rank order of importance

Females	Deaths
1. Tuberculosis	329
2.Pneumonia	242
3. Heart Disease	164
4. Gastrointestinal	65
5. Cancer	58
Influenza	58
Meningitis	58
8. Stroke	30
9. Premature Birth	26
10. Natural Causes	24
11. Childbirth	23
Total	**1,077**

Males	Deaths
1. Pneumonia	323
2. Tuberculosis	289
3. Heart Disease	158
4. Misc. Accidents	114
5. Auto Accidents	71
6. Gastrointestinal	59
7. Influenza	46
8. Premature Birth	38
9. Alcohol Related	28
10. Cancer	24
Total	**1,150**

Figure 3.12. Crude death rates for Yakama, white,
& non-white U. S. populations

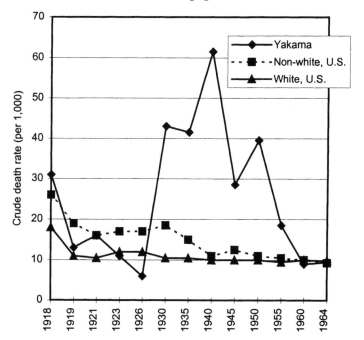

Figure 3.13. Yakama heart disease deaths by age group and gender

Age	Female	Row %	Male	Row %	Total
<5	11	55	8	40	19
5-9	3	100	0	0	3
10-14	3	60	2	40	5
15-19	0	0	0	0	0
20-24	0	0	4	100	4
25-29	4	80	1	20	5
30-34	1	50	1	50	2
35-39	11	85	2	15	13
40-44	3	23	10	77	13
45-49	8	44	10	56	18
50-54	10	63	6	37	16
55-59	11	42	14	54	25
60-64	11	35	20	65	31
65-69	16	46	19	54	35
70-74	17	50	20	63	37
75-79	17	50	17	50	34
>80	42	65	23	35	65
Total	168		157		325

Note: Table excludes cases missing on age and gender

Figure 3.14. Yakama gastrointestinal deaths
by gender and age group

Age	Female	Row %	Male	Row %	Total
<5	51	49	54	51	105
5-9	2	67	1	33	3
10-14	0	0	0	0	0
15-19	1	100	0	0	1
20-24	0	0	0	0	0
25-29	0	0	1	100	1
30-34	3	100	0	0	3
35-39	0	0	0	0	0
40-44	1	100	0	0	1
45-49	0	0	0	0	0
50-54	0	0	0	0	0
55-59	1	100	0	0	1
60-64	1	100	0	0	1
65-69	1	100	0	0	1
70-74	1	100	0	0	1
75-79	3	100	0	0	3
>80	0	0	3	100	3
Total	65		59		124

Note: Table excludes cases missing on age and gender

Figure 3.15. Moving averages for Yakama gastrointestinal disorders

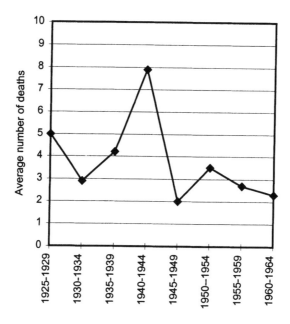

Figure 3.16. Leading causes of death by blood quantum

Cause	Full	Row %	Half	Row %	Quarter	Row %	Total
Tuberculosis	394	80	57	12	41	8	492
Pneumonia	309	84	43	12	14	4	366
Heart Disease	108	70	34	22	13	8	155
Misc. Accidents	62	74	11	13	11	13	84
Gastrointestinal	49	73	14	21	4	6	67
Cancer	22	58	8	21	8	21	38
Premature Birth	25	74	5	15	4	11	34
Auto Accidents	36	86	4	10	2	4	42
Influenza	90	97	1	1	2	2	93
Senility	53	98	0	0	1	2	54
Total	1,148		177		100		1,425

Figure 4.1. Yakama population data

Year	Births	Deaths	Population	Year	Births	Deaths	Population
1885			1,272	1927	19	157	3,025
1887			1,741	1928	57	229	2,974
1888		1	1,765	1929	73	139	2,955
1889			1,675	1930	55	181	2,908
1890		1	1,406	1931	83	158	2,916
1891			2,311	1932	95	129	2,971
1893			1,308	1933	91	115	3,026
1894			1,927	1934	83	120	3,081
1895		1	1,808	1935	89	89	3,136
1896			1,821	1936	63	107	3,191
1897			1,792	1937	60	113	3,246
1898			2,356	1938	81	61	3,301
1899		1	2,343	1939	72	144	3,356.
1900		1	2,309	1940	79	132	3,411
1901		1	2,311	1941	87	108	3,466
1902			2,300	1942	92	68	3,521
1903			2,302	1943	119	86	3,576
1904			2,291	1944	103	93	3,631
1905			2,300	1945	107	65	3,686
1906		3	2,001	1946	80	42	3,741
1907			2,002	1947	88	39	3,796
1908		1		1948	106	34	3,851
1909	11	1		1949	103	46	3,906
1910		6	2,679	1950	72	29	3,961
1911		68	2,622	1951	62	24	4,016
1912		4	3,046	1953	128	41	4,071
1913		2	3,052	1953	96	42	4,126
1914	2	23	3,149	1954	135	52	4,181
1915	5	37	3,146	1955	120	54	4,236
1916	4	28	3,086	1956	129	37	4,300
1917	7	21	3,000	1957	130	43	4,436
1918	7	94	3,000	1958	151	48	4,572
1919	8	40	2,927	1959	162	42	4,708
1920	9	47	2,910	1960	205	39	4,844
1921	13	33	2,893	1961	174	40	4,981
1922	17	24	2,955	1962	186	59	5,118
1923	7	16	2,934	1963	144	53	5,313
1924	8	80	2,982	1964	230	46	5,508
1925	6	133	3,001	1965			5,703
1926	8	128	3,032	1980			6,856

Note: Population figures for the years 1885 through 1931 are based on Yakama tribal censuses; figures for the years from 1932 through 1964 are estimates, except for the years 1956, 1960, 1962, and 1965

Figure 4.2. Resident population of the
United States for selected years

1919	104,514,000
1926	117,397,000
1930	123,077,000
1935	127,250,000
1940	131,954,000
1945	132,481,000
1950	151,235,000
1955	164,308,000
1960	179,979,000
1964	191,141,000

Source: *Historical Statistics of the United States: Colonial Times to 1970*

Figure 4.3. Resident population of
Washington, selected years

1920	1,367,000
1926	1,488,000
1930	1,563,396
1935	1,629,000
1940	1,736,191
1945	2,206,000
1950	2,378,763
1955	2,604,000
1960	2,853,214

Source: *Statistical Abstracts of the United States,* United States Department of Commerce

Figure 4.4. Comparative rates (per 100,000) for leading causes
at ten-year intervals

	1910	1920	1930	1940	1950	1960
Tuberculosis						
Yakama	na	34	1,428	868	76	na
African American	446	262	192	128	52	13
White	146	100	58	37	18	5
United States	154	113	71	46	23	6
Pneumonia						
Yakama	na	na	850	644	125	133
African American	92	28	12	10	49	54
White	50	8	3	3	24	30
United States	156	207	103	70	31	40
Heart Disease						
Yakama	na	34	238	224	125	171
African American	205	161	225	249	310	287
White	158	160	213	298	361	380
United States	372	365	414	486	356	522
Misc. Accidents						
Yakama	na	34	204	112	na	171
African American	92	73	64	52	47	44
White	83	60	63	46	36	29
United States	82	60	54	47	38	31
Gastrointestinal						
Yakama	na	na	170	420	na	na
African American	na	na	na	na	24	na
White	na	na	na	na	16	na
United States	115	54	26	10	17	4
Auto Accidents						
Yakama	na	34	na	140	25	na
African American	1	5	22	24	24	22
White	2	11	27	25	23	21
United States	76	83	97	120	23	149
Influenza						
Yakama	na	34	na	84	na	na
African American	16	108	38	33	10	8
White	14	67	17	13	4	4
United States	156	207	103	70	31	37
Cancer						
Yakama	na	na	na	84	76	19
African American	54	49	57	78	108	122
White	77	87	102	97	144	153
United States	76	83	97	120	140	149

Note: Rates for influenza and pneumonia are combined for the United States.

Figure 4.5. Leading causes of Yakama death, 1950-1964

Cause	Deaths	Percentage
Heart disease	127	35.0%
Pneumonia	125	34.7%
Auto accidents	62	17.0%
Cancer	33	9.0%

Figure 4.6. Leading types of Yakama cancer deaths by gender

Type	Female	Row %	Male	Row %	Total
Uterine	17	100%	na	0%	17
Stomach	14	78%	4	22%	18
Breast	9	100%	0	0%	9
Cervical	4	100%	na	0%	4
Prostate	na	0%	4	100%	4
Bladder	0	0%	3	100%	3
Lung	2	40%	3	60%	5
Liver	4	67%	2	33%	6
Other	8	50%	8	50%	16
Total	58		24		82

Figure 4.7. Moving averages for Yakama Heart Disease

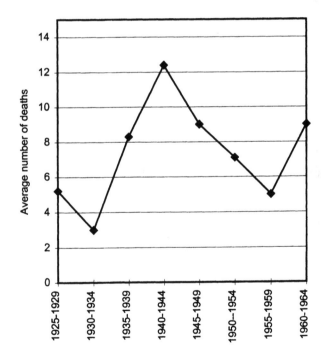

Figure 4.8. Leading causes of death among
Yakama children, 1888-1964

Under 1 year of age	1 year of age	2 to 5 years of age
1. Pneumonia	1. Pneumonia	1. Pneumonia
2. Gastrointestinal	2. Gastrointestinal	2. Tuberculosis
3. Tuberculosis	3. Tuberculosis	3. Gastrointestinal
4. Heart disease	4. Misc. accidents	4. Meningitis
5. Syphilis	5. Whooping cough	5. Misc. accidents

Figure 4.9. Fetal death rates: Yakama, white U.S., and non-white U.S.

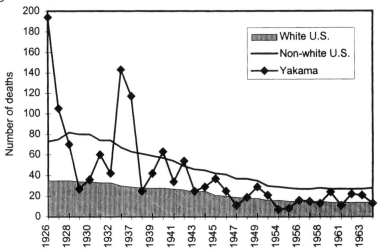

Figure 4.10. Cause of death by gender for Yakama under
one year of age, 1888-1964

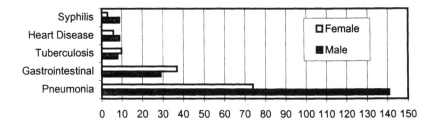

Figure 4.11. Infant mortality rate
averages per 1,000 live births

Years	Yakama	White	Non-white	State of Washington
1920-1924	253	74	113	59
1925-1929	497	65	105	51
1930-1934	331	56	93	45
1935-1939	225	49	81	41
1940-1944	232	39	67	34
1945-1949	81	31	50	30
1950-1954	86	26	45	25
1955-1959	80	23	44	23
1960-1964	52	22	42	22

Figure 4.12. Comparative infant mortality rates (moving averages)

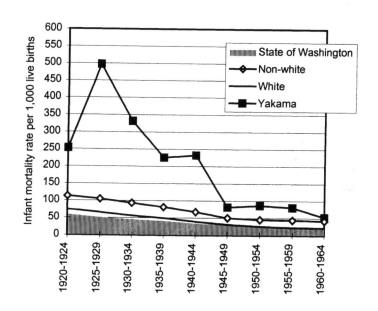

Figure 4.13. Moving averages, fetal deaths
per 1,000 live births, 1920-1964

Years	Yakama	White	Non-white
1926-1929	99	35	78
1930-1934	46	33	76
1935-1939	82	29	63
1940-1944	41	26	50
1945-1949	24	19	39
1950-1954	14	16	30
1955-1959	13	15	28
1960-1964	18	14	27

Figure 5.1. Yakama crude death rates for selected years

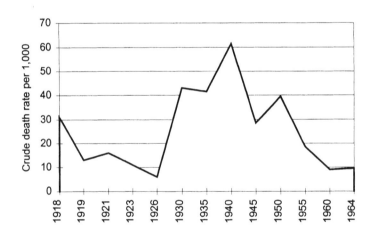

BIBLIOGRAPHY

Manuscript Collections

Click Relander Collection, Yakima Valley Regional Library, Yakima, Washington.

Dean and Geraldine Guie Collection, Yakima, Washington: Mourning Dove's autobiographical manuscript and traditional stories.

Department of Native American Studies, University of California, Riverside, California: Birkby, George, Jim, Jones, Kamiakin, Nightwalker, Patrick, Peone Interviews; Bartlett, Scheuerman, and Seeman Manuscripts; Palouse Indian Calendar; Kamiakin Geneaology.

Granville O. Haller Collection, Bancroft Library, University of California, Berkeley.

Lucullus Virgil McWhorter Collection, Manuscripts, Archives, and Special Collections, Washington State University, Pullman, Washington.

National Archives, Pacific Northwest, Seattle, Washington: Yakima Agency Records, Death Certificates, Agency Letterbooks, Birth Records.

National Archives, Washington, D.C.: Records of the Bureau of Indian Affairs, War Department, State Department, Indian Claims Commission.

William Compton Brown Collection, Manuscripts Archives and Special Collections, Washington State University, Pullman, Washington.

World Population Data Sheet, Population Reference Bureau, Inc., Washington, D. C., 1983.

Original Sources

Allen, Paul. *History of the Expedition Under the Command of Captains Lewis and Clark*. London: Longman, Hurst, Rees, Orme, and Brown, 1814.

Annual Reports of the Commissioners of Indian Affairs. Washington, D. C.: Government Printing Office.

Ault, Nelson A., ed. *The Papers of Lucullus Virgil McWhorter*. Pullman, Washington: Washington State College, 1959.

Benson, Todd. "Race, Health, and Power: The Federal Government and American Indian Health, 1909-1965." Ph. D. dissertation. Stanford: Stanford University, 1993.

Bischoff, William N. "The Yakima Indian War: 1855-1856." Ph. D. dissertation, Loyola University of Chicago, 1950.

Blanchet, Francis Norbert. *Historical Sketches of the Catholic Church of Oregon*. Portland, Oregon: Catholic Sentinel, 1878.

Boyd, Robert T. "The Introduction of Infectious Diseases among the Indians of the Pacific Northwest, 1774-1874." Ph.D dissertation, University of Washington, Seattle, 1985.

Brown, William Compton. *The Indian Side of the Story*. Spokane: C. W. Hill Printing Company, 1961.

Bureau of Indian Affairs, *Report on the Source, Nature and Extent of Fishing, Hunting and Miscellaneous Related Rights of Certain Tribes in Oregon and Washington*. . . . (Los Angeles: Office of Indian Affairs, Division of Forestry and Grazing, 1942).

California Area 1993 Profile. Sacramento: California Area Office, Indian Health Service, 1994.

Chalfant, Stewart. "Ethno-historical Report on Aboriginal Land Occupancy and Utilization by the Palus Indians." Defense Exhibit 69, United States Indian Claims Commission, National Archives, Record Group 279.

Chittenden, H. M. and A. T. Richardson, eds. *Life, Letters and Travels of Father Pierre Jean DeSmet, S. J., 1801-1873: Missionary Labors and Adventures Among the Wild Tribes of the North American Indians, Embracing Minute Descriptions of their Manners, Customs, Modes of Warfare and Torture.* . . . . 4 Volumes, New York: Francis P. Harper, 1905.

Clayman, Charles B., ed. *The American Medical Association Enclyclopedia of Medicine.* New York: Random House, 1989.

Coan, Charles F. "Federal Indian Policy in the Pacific Northwest, 1849- 1870." Ph. D. dissertation, University of California, 1920.

Cox, Ross. *Adventures on the Columbia River.* 2 Volumes. London: H. Colburn and R. Bentley, 1831. Reprinted in 1957 by the University of Oklahoma Press as The Columbia River.

Curtis, Edward S. *Indian Days of the Long Ago.* New York: World Book Company, 1915.

_____. *The North American Indians.* Norwood, Massachusetts: Plimpton Press, 1911.

DeSmet, Pierre Jean. *Oregon Missions and Travels Over the Rocky Mountains in 1845-46.* New York: Edward Dunigan, 1847.

_____. *Origin, Progress and Prospects of the Catholic Mission to the Rocky Mountains.* Philadelphia: M. Fithian, 1843.

Documents Relating to Negotiations of Ratified and Unratified Treaties. National Archives, Record Group 75. Microfilm T 494, Reel 5.

"Doty's Journal of Operations." Documents Relating to Negotiations of Ratified and Unratified Treaties. National Archives, Record Group 75. Microfilm T494. Reel 5.

DuBois, Cora. "The Feather Cult of the Middle Columbia." *General Series in Anthropology 7.* Menasha, Wisconsin: The George Banta Publishing Company, 1938.

Elliott, T. C., ed. "David Thompson's Journeys in the Spokane Country." *Washington Historical Quarterly* 8 (1917: 183-187, 261-264; 9 (1918): 11-16, 103-106, 169-173, 284-887; 10 (1919): 17-20.

_____. "Journal of David Thompson." *Oregon Historical Quarterly* 15 (1914): 39-63, 104-25.

Franchere, Gabriel. *Narrative of A Voyage To the Northwest Coast of America In the Years 1811, 1812, 1813, and 1814, Or the First American Settlement on the Pacific.* New York: Redfield, 1854.

Gibbs, George, et al. "Report on the Indian Tribes of the Territory of Washington." *Secretary of War Reports of Explorations* 1 (1854): 400- 449: [see *House Executive Document* 91, 33rd Cong. 1st Sess. and Reprinted in 1972 by Ye Galleon Press, Fairfield, Washington.

Gibbs, George. "Tribes of Western Washington and Northwestern Oregon Published with Extensive Vocabularies," in W. H. Dall, Tribes of the Extreme Northwest, *Contributions to North American Ethnology*, 1, for United States Geographical and Geological Survey of the Rocky Mountain Region. J. W. Powell, Director, Washington, D.C., 1877: 163-361.

Gilbert, Frank T. *Historic Sketches of Walla Walla, Whitman, Columbia and Garfield Counties, Washington Territory*. Portland, Oregon: A. G. Walling Co., 1882.

Haller, Granville O. "Kamiakin--In History: Memoir of the War, in the Yakima Valley, 1855-1856." Manuscript A128, Bancroft Library, University of California, Berkeley.

Holy Bible. New York: Oxford University Press, 1973.

Howard, Oliver O. *My Life and Experiences Among Our Hostile Indians: A Report of Personal Observations, Adventures, and Campaigns Among the Indians of the Great West, With some Account of Their Life, Habits, Traits, Religion, Ceremonies, Dress, Savage Instincts, and Customs in Peace and War*. Hartford: A. D. Worthington and Co., 1907.

_____. *Nez Perce Joseph*. Boston: Lee and Sheperd, 1881.

Hunter, George. *Reminiscences of an Old Timer*. San Francisco: H. S. Crocker and Co., 1887.

Indian Claims Commission. "Evidence in Support of Proposed Findings of Fact of Petitioners in Docket Number 222 on Issues of Liability." United States Claims Commission. National Archives, Record Group 279.

_____. "Testimony of Verne L. Ray." United States Claims Commission. National Archives, Record Group 279.

Indian Claims Commission Decisions. Volume 7, Part B and Volume 12, Part A. Boulder, Colorado: Native American Rights Fund, n.d.

Indian Health Service. Trends in Indian Health, 1991. Washington, D. C.: United States Department of Health and Human Services, 1991.

Jim, Mary. "A Palouse Indian Speaks." *The Bunchgrass Historian* 8 (1980): 20-23.

Johansen, Dorothy C., ed. *Robert Newell's Memoranda.* Portland, Oregon: Champoeg Press, 1959.

Kappler, Charles J. *Indian Affairs, Laws and Treaties.* 2 Volumes. Washington, D. C.: Government Printing Office, 1940.

Keeley, Patrick. "Nutrient Composition of Selected Important Plant Foods of the Precontact Diet of the Northwestern Native American Peoples." Master's thesis, University of Washington, Seattle, 1980.

Kip, Lawrence. *Army Life on the Pacific: A Journal of the Expedition Against the Northern Indians, the Tribes of the Coeur d'Alenes, Spokanes, and Pelouzes, in the Summer of 1858.* New York: Redfield Publishing Co., 1859.

Koenig, Margaret W. *Tuberculosis Among the Nebraska Winnebago: A Social Study on an Indian Reservation.* Lincoln: Nebraska State Historical Society, 1921.

Kuykendall, G. B. "Spirit Beliefs." Unpublished manuscript. Relander Collection, Yakima Valley Regional Library.

Langone, Stephen A. "A Statistical Profile of the Indian: The Lack of Numbers." *United States Congress, Joint Economic Committee, Toward Economic Development for Native American Communities.* Vol. 2. Washiangton D.C.: United States Government Printing Office, 1969.

Manual X: Indirect Techniques for Demographic Estimations. New York: Department of International Economic and Social Affairs, Population Studies, Number 81, United Nations, 1983.

McWhorter, LuceullusVirgil. *Hear Me, My Chiefs!* Caldwell, Idaho: The Caxton Printers, Ltd., 1952.

_____. *Tragedy of the Whak-Shum; Prelude to the Yakima Indian War, 1855-56*: The Killing of Major Andrew J. Bolon. Fairfield, Washington: Ye Galleon Press, 1958.

Masterson, James R. "The Records of the Washington Superintendency of Indian Affairs, 1853-1874." *Pacific Northwest Quarterly* 37 (1946): 31-41.

Meriam, Lewis. *The Problem of Indian Administration.* New York: The Johnson Reprint Corporation, 1971.

Merk, Frederick, ed. *Fur Trade and Empire: George Simpson's Journal, 1824-1825.* Cambridge, Massachusetts: Belknap Press, 1968.

Mermel, T.W., ed. and comp. *Register of Dams in the United States: Completed, Under Construction and Proposed.* New York: McGraw Hill, 1958.

Mooney, James. "The Ghost Dance Religion and the Sioux Outbreak of 1890." *Fourteenth Annual Report to the Bureau of American Ethnology,* Washington, D. C.: Government Printing Office, 1892-1893.

Moran, John, and Evelyn Broncheau, Corky Covington, Pam Garza, Sharon John, Jim Horst, Linda Kafford, Karen Schmidt, and Jim Sutherland, Yakima Indian Health Center Morbidity and Mortality Committee. "1991 Mortality Report." Toppenish, Washington: Yakima Indian Health Center, Yakima Nation, 1992.

Morton, Arthur S., ed. "The North West Company's Columbia Enterprise and David Thompson." *Canadian Historical Review* 17 (1936): 266-288; 18 (1937): 156-162.

Moulton, Gary, ed. *Journals of Lewis and Clark.* 7 Volumes. Lincoln: University of Nebraska Press, 1983-1990.

Mullan, John. *Report on the Construction of a Military Road from Fort Walla Walla to Fort Benton.* Washington, D. C.: Government Printing Office, 1863.

_____. "Report on the Indian Tribes in the Eastern Portion of Washington Territory, 1853." *Secretary of War, Reports of Explorations* 1, 437- 441.

_____. "Topographical Memoir and Map of Colonel Wright's Late Campaign Against the Indians of Oregon and Washington Territories." *Senate Executive Document,* 35th Congress, 2nd Session, No. 32, SS 984.

"New, Reemerging, and Drug Resistant Infections." *Home Page. National Center for Infectious Diseases.* Atlanta: Center for Disease Control, 1996.

Official Register of the United States, 1883. Washington, D. C.: United States Government Printing Office, 1889.

_____, 1889. Washington, D. C.: United States Government Prinnting Office, 1891.

_____, 1893. Washington, D. C.: United States Government Printing Office, 1893.

_____, 1895. Washington, D. C.: United States Government Printing Office, 1895.

_____, 1897. Washington, D. C.: United States Government Printing Office, 1897.

Pambrun, Andrew D. *Sixty Years on the Frontier in the Pacific Northwest.* Edward J. Kowrach, ed. Fairfield, Washington: Ye Galleon Press, 1978.

Putney, Diane T. "Fighting the Scourge: American Indian Morbidity and Federal Policy, 1897-1930." Ph. D. dissertation. Milwaukee: Marquette University, 1980.

Puyallup Tribe v. Department of Game. United States Supreme Court, 1968.

Quaife, Milo Milton. *Adventures of the First Settlers on the Oregon or Columbia River.* Chicago: The Lakeside Press, 1923.

Ray, Verne F. "Economic Use of the Tribal Territory of the Yakima," United States Indian Claims Commission, Dockets 47 and 47A, National Archives, Record Group 279.

Regional Differences in Indian Health. Washington, D. C.: United States Department of Health, Indian Health Service, 1993.

Relander, Click. "Sophie Williams' Interview in Colville and Palouse Notes." Unpublished manuscript. Relander Collection. Yakima Valley Regional Library.

Ross, Alexander. *Adventures of the First Settlers on the Oregon or Columbia River: Being a Narrative of the Expedition Fitted Out by John Jacob Astor to Establish the "Pacific Fur Company"; With an Account of Some Indian Tribes on the Coast of the Pacific.* London: Smith, Elder and Company, 1849.

_____. *The Fur Hunters of the Far West; A Narrative of Adventures in the Oregon and Rocky Mountains.* Norman: University of Oklahoma Press, 1956.

Schmeckebier, Laurence F. *The Office of Indian Affairs: Its History, Activities, and Organization.* Institute for Government Research, Service Monographs of the United States, No. 48. Baltimore: The Johns Hopkins Press, 1927.

Schoolcraft, Henry Rowe. *Historical and Statistical Information Respecting the History, Conditions, and Prospects of the Indian Tribes of the United States.* 6 volumes. Philadelphia: Lippincott, Grambo, and Company, 1851-1857.

Schuster, Helen H. "Yakima Indian Traditionalism: A Study in Continuity and Change." Ph. D. dissertation, University of Washington, Seattle, 1975.

Secretary of War, *Reports of Explorations and Surveys to Ascertain the Most Practicable and Economical Route for a Railroad from the Mississippi River to the Pacific Ocean, Made Under the Direction of the Secretary of War, in 1853-55.* 12 Volumes. Washington, D.C.: Government Printing Office, 1855-60.

Sharkey, Margery. "Revitalization and Change: A History of the Wanapum Indians, Their Prophet Smowhala, and the Washani Religion." Master's thesis, Washington State University, Pullman, 1984.

Sohappy v. Smith. United States Supreme Court, 1969.

Sprague, Roderick. "Aboriginal Burial Practices in the Plateau Region of North America." Ph. D. dissertation, University of Arizona, Tucson, 1967.

Stevens, Hazard. *The Life of Issac Ingalls Stevens.* 2 Volumes. Boston: Houghton, Mifflin and Company, 1901.

Stewart, W. M. "David Thompson's Surveys in the North-West." *Canadian Historical Review* 17 (1936).

Stuart, Paul. *Nations Within A Nation: Historical Statistics of American Indians.* New York: Greenwood Press, 1987.

_____. "The Indian Office: Growth and Development of an American Institution, 1865-1900." *Studies in American History and Culture,* No. 12. Ann Arbor: UMI Research Press, 1979.

Trafzer, Clifford E. *Grandmother, Grandfather, and Old Wolf.* East Lansing: Michigan State University Press, forthcoming, 1997.

"Tuberculosis." *Med Facts.* Denver: National Jewish Center for Immunology and Respiratory Medicine, 1987.

"Tuberculosis Among the North American Indians." *Report of a Committee of the National Tuberculosis Association Appointed on October 28, 1921 on Tuberculosis Among the North American Indians.* Washington, D. C.: United States Government Printing Office, 1923.

Uncommon Controversy. A Report Prepared for the American Friends Service Committee. Seattle: University of Washington Press, 1970.

United States Bureau of Census. Census, Ninth through Fourteenth, 1870- 1920.

_____. Census of Population: 1950. *Characteristics of the Population, United States* Summary 12, pt. 1. Washington, D. C.: United States Government Printing Office, 1953.

_____. Census of Population 1950: Special Reports. *Non-white Population by Race. P-E No. 3B.* Washington, D. C.: United States Government Printing Office, 1953.

_____. Census of Population: 1960. *Characteristics of the Population, United States* Summary 1, pt. 1. Washington. D.C.: United States Government Printing Office, 1964.

_____. Census of Population: 1960. *Special Reports. Non-white Population by Race.* Final Report PC [2]-1C. Washington, D. C.: United States Government Printing Office, 1963.

_____. *Report on Indians Taxed and Indians Not Taxed in the United States (Excluding Alaska) at the Eleventh Census: 1890.* Washington, D. C.: United States Government Printing Office, 1894.

_____. *The Indian Population of the United States and Alaska: 1930.* Washington D.C.: United States Government Printing Office, 1937.

United States Commissioners of Indian Affairs, *Annual Reports,* 1824-1949. Reprinted by Microcard Editions. Washington, D. C., 1968.

United States Congress, House of Representatives, Committee on Interior and Insular Affairs. *Investigation of the Bureau of Indian Affairs.* 82nd Congress, 2nd Session, House Reports, No. 2503, SS 11582. Washington, D. C.: United States Government Printing Office, 1953.

United States Department of the Army. *Review Report on Columbia River and Tributaries.* North Pacific Division Corps of Engineers, 1948.

United States Department of Commerce. *Historical Statistics of the United States: Colonial Times to 1970.* Washington, D. C.: Department of Commerce, 1975.

_____. *The Social and Economic Status of the Black Population in the United States. An Historical View, 1790-1978.* Washington, D. C.: Department of Commerce, 1978. United States v Washington . United States Supreme Court, 1974..

United States Department of Health and Human Services. *Trends and Current Status in Childhood Mortality: United States, 1900-1985.* Washington, D. C.: Public Health Service, Center for Disease Control, 1985.

United States Department of Interior. "The Columbia River." *House Executive Document 473,* 81st Congress, 2nd Session, 1950.

_____. *The Indian Population of the United States and Alaska.* Washington, D. C.: United States Government Printing Office, 1917.

United States Indian Health Service. *Chart Series Book, April 1986.* Washington, D. C.: United States Government Printing Office, 1986.

United States Public Health Service. *Whooping Cough.* Washington, D. C.: Public Health Service, 1957.

Washington Territorial Census, 1871. National Archives. Microfilm 276, Reel 8.

Winthrop, Theodore. *The Canoe and the Saddle or Klalam and Klickitat.* Tacoma, Washington: John H. Williams, 1913.

Yakima Tribal Council. *The Yakimas: Treaty Centennial, 1855-1955.* Yakima, Washington: Republic Press, 1955.

Oral Interviews, Correspondence, Video

Andrew George to Clifford E. Trafzer, May 29, 1987.

Clifford E. Trafzer with John Moran, M. D., May 4, 1993, Yakama Indian Reservation, Telephone Communication.

_____ with Mary Nelson, 1988, Olympia, Washington.

_____ with James Sandos, April 4, May 22, 1995, Redlands, California.

_____ and Richard D. Scheuerman with Mary Jim, May 1, 1977; April 2 and November 10, 17, 1979; April 25, 1980, Yakama Indian Reservation.

_____, Richard D. Scheuerman, and Lee Ann Smith with Andrew George, November 15, 1981, Yakama Indian Reservation.

_____ with Brad Richie, M. D., May 18, 1993, Colton, California.

_____ with Kirsten Holm, Washington Center for Health Research, April 3, 1994, Telephone Communication.

_____ with Lee Francis, Bureau of Indian Affairs, April 3, 1994, Telephone Communication.

Craig Leslie. Photograph of Andrew George leading a Washani Funeral, Portland, Oregon.

Eugene S. Hunn to Clifford E. Trafzer, May 18, 1994.

John R. Weeks to Clifford E. Trafzer, June 15, 1994.

Lisa Firth to Clifford E. Trafzer, December 1, 1992.

Richard D. Scheuerman with Emily Peone, January-May, 1981, Colville Indian Reservation.

_____ with Geraldine Guie, 1983, Yakima, Washington.

Video of Ida Nason, "Everything Changing, Everything Changing," University of Washington.

Newspapers

Los Angeles Times, May 7-8, 1995.
San Bernardino Sun, March 15, 1994.
Spokesman Review, August 13, 1936.

Books

Armstrong, A. N. *Oregon: Comprising A Brief History and Full Descriptions of the Territories of Oregon and Washington.* Chicago: C. Scott and Company, 1857.

Bakeless, John. *Lewis and Clark, Partners in Discovery.* New York: W. Morrow, 1947.

Ballou, Robert. *Early Klickitat Valley Days.* Goldendale, Washington: Goldendale Sentinel, 1938.

Bancroft, Hubert Howe. *History of Oregon.* San Francisco: The History Company, 1888.

_____. *History of the Northwest Coast.* San Francisco: A. L. Bancroft and Company. 1884.

_____. *History of Washington, Idaho and Montana.* San Francisco: The History Company, 1890.

_____. *Native Races of the Pacific States of North America.* San Francisco: The History Company, 1886.

Barnett, Homer G. *Indian Shakers: A Messianic Cult of the Pacific Northwest.* Carbondale: Southern Illinois University Press, 1972.

Bates, Barbara. *Bargaining for Life: A Social History of Tuberculosis, 1876-1938.* Philadelphia: University of Pennsylvania Press, 1992.

Beavert, Virginia, ed., *The Way It Was: Anaku Iwacha.* Toppenish, Washington: Franklin Press, 1974.

Berreman, Joel V. "Tribal Distribution in Oregon." *American Anthropological Association Memoir* 47. Menasha, Wisconsin, 1937.

Brown, William J., James F. Donohue, Norman W. Axnick, Joseph H. Blount, Neal H. Ewen, and Oscar G. Jones. *Syphilis and Other Venereal Diseases.* Cambridge: Harvard University Press, 1970.

Burnet, Frank MacFarlan and David O. White. *Natural History of Infectious Diseases.* Cambridge: Cambridge University Press, 1972.

Burns, Robert Ignatius. *The Jesuits and the Indian Wars of the Northwest.* New Haven: Yale University Press, 1966.

Cannon, Miles. *Waiilatpu, Its Rise and Fall, 1836-1847; A Story of Pioneer Days in the Pacific Northwest.* Boise, Idaho: Capital News Job Rooms, 1915.

Caputi, Jane. *Gossips, Gorgons & Crones: The Fates of the Earth.* Santa Fe: Bear & Company, 1993.

Cartwright, Frederick Fox. *Disease and History.* London: Hart-Davis, 1972.

Chalfant, Stuart. *Interior Salish and Eastern Washington Indians.* New York: Garland Publishing, 1974.

Christie, Andrew B. *Infectious Diseases: Epidemiology and Clinical Practice.* Edinburgh and London: E. and S. Livingstone, 1969.

Chuinard, E. G. *The Medical Aspects of the Lewis and Clark Expedition.* Corvallis, Oregon: Oregon State University Friends of the Library, 1954.

Clark, Ella. *Indian Legends of the Pacific Northwest.* Berkeley: University of California Press, 1953.

Cohen, Felix S. *Handbook of Federal Indian Law.* Albuquerque: University of New Mexico Press, 1971.

Collins, Selwyn Dewitt and Josephine Lehmann. *Excess Deaths from Influenza and Pneumonia and from Important Chronic Diseases During Epidemic Periods, 1918-1951.* Washington, D. C.: Public Health Service, 1953.

Cook, Sherburne F. *The Conflict Between the California Indian and White Civilization.* Berkeley: University of California Press, 1976.

_____. *The Population of the California Indians, 1769-1970.* Berkeley: University of California Press, 1976.

Corner, Beryl Dorothy. *Prematurity: The Diagnosis, Care and Disorders of the Premature Infant.* London: Cassell, 1960.

Cox, Ross. *The Columbia River.* Norman: University of Oklahoma Press, 1957.

Crosby, Alfred W. *Ecological Imperialism: The Biological Expansion of Europe, 900-1900.* Cambridge: Cambridge University Press, 1986.

_____. *The Columbian Exchange: Biological and Cultural Consequences of 1492.* Westport, Connecticut: Greenwood Publishing Company, 1972.

Culverwell, Albert. *Stronghold in the Yakima Country.* Olympia, Washington: Washington State Parks and Recreation Commission, 1956.

Desmond, G. B. *Gambling Among the Yakimas.* Washington, D. C.: Catholic University of America Press, 1952.

Dobyns, Henry F. *Native American Historical Demography: A Critical Bibliography.* Bloomington: Indiana University Press, 1976.

_____. *Their Number Became Thinned: Native American Population Dynamics in Eastern North America*. Knoxville: University of Tennessee Press, 1983.

Drury, Clifford M. *Marcus Whitman*. Caldwell, Idaho: The Caxton Printers, Ltd., 1936.

_____. *Marcus Whitman, M.D.: Pioneer and Martyr*. Caldwell, Idaho: The Caxton Printers, Ltd., 1937.

_____. *Tepee In His Front Yard*. Portland, Oregon: Binfords and Mort, 1949.

Dubos, René and Jean Dubos. *The White Plague: Tuberculosis, Man, and Society*. Boston: Little, Brown & Company, 1952. Reprinted in 1992 by Rutgers University Press, New Brunswick, New Jersey.

Getches, David H. and Charles F. Wilkinson. *Federal Indian Law*. St. Paul, Minnesota: West Publishing Company, 1986.

Gibbs, George. *Indian Tribes of Washington Territory*. Fairfield, Washington: Ye Galleon Press, 1972.

Gibson, Arrell M. *The American Indian: Prehistory to Present*. Lexington, Massachusetts: D. C. Heath, 1980.

Gidley, M. *With One Sky Above Us*. Seattle: University of Washington Press, 1974.

Gilbert, Frank T. *The Whitman Massacre, With a Few Prior Historical Events*. Portland, Oregon: North Pacific History Company, 1888.

Guie, H. Dean. *Bugles in the Valley: The Story of Garnett's Fort Simcoe*. Portland: Oregon Historical Society, 1977.

Heizer, Robert F. *California*. Washington, D. C.: Smithsonian Institution Press, 1978.

Hess, Julius H. and Evelyn C. Lundeen. *The Premature Infant*. Philadelphia: Lippincott, 1949.

Hines, Donald M. *Magic in the Mountains. The Yakima Shaman: Power and Practice*. Issaquah, Washington: Great Eagle Publishing, 1993.

Hodge, Frederick W., ed. *Handbook of American Indians North of Mexico*. 2 Volumes. Washington, D.C.: United States Government Printing Office, 1907-1910.

Hoopes, A. W. *Indian Affairs and their Administration, 1849-1860, With Especial Reference to the Far West.* Philadelphia: University of Pennsylvania Press, 1932.

Howard, Cheryl. *Navajo Tribal Demography, 1983-1986: A Comparative and Historical Perspective.* New York: Garland, 1993.

Hull, Lindley M. *A History of Central Washington, Including the Famous Wenatchee, Entiat, Chelan and Columbia Valleys.* Spokane: Shaw and Borden Company, 1932.

Hultkrantz, Ake. *Conceptions of the Soul Among North American Indians.* Stockholm: The Ethnographical Museum of Sweden, 1953.

_____. *The North American Indian Orpheus Tradition.* Stockholm: The Ethnographical Museum of Sweden, 1957.

Hunn, Eugene S. with James Selam. *Nch'i-Wana, "The Big River": Mid-Columbia Indians and Their Land.* Seattle: University of Washington Press, 1990.

Johansen, Dorothy O. and Charles M. Gates. *Empire of the Columbia: A History of the Pacific Northwest.* New York: Harper & Row, 1967.

Josephy, Alvin M., Jr., *The Nez Perce Indians and the Opening of the Northwest.* New Haven: Yale University Press, 1965.

Kimmel, Thelma. *The Fort Simcoe Story.* Toppenish, Washington: The Toppenish Review, 1954.

Kuntz, Jeffrey and Asher J. Finkle. *The American Medical Association Family Medical Guide.* New York: Random House, 1987.

Kvasnicka, Robert M. and Herman J. Viola, eds. *The Commissioners of Indian Affairs.* Lincoln: University of Nebraska Press, 1979.

La Barre, Weston. *Ghost Dance: Origins of Religion.* New York: Dell Publishing Company, 1972.

Lapin, Joseph H. *Whooping Cough.* Springfield, Illinois: C. C. Thomas, 1943.

Lebenthan, Emanuel, ed. *Textbook of Gastroenterology and Nutrition in Infancy.* New York: Raven Press, 1981.

Lundeen, Evelyn C. and Ralph H. Kunstadter. *Care of the Premature Infant.* Philadelphia: Lippincott, 1958.

Lyman, W. D. *History of the Yakima Valley, Washington, Comprising Yakima, Kittitas and Benton Counties.* Chicago: S. J. Clarke, 1919.

Lynn, William S. *Inflammatory Cells and Lung Disease.* Boca Raton, Florida: CRC Press, 1983.

McKeown, Thomas. *The Modern Rise of Population.* New York: Academic Press, 1976.

McNeil, William H. *Plagues and People.* Garden City: Anchor Doubleday, 1976.

McWhorter, Lucullus Virgil. *The Crime Against the Yakima.* North Yakima, Washington: Republic Press, 1913.

Manypenny, George W. *Our Indian Wards.* New York: Da Capo Press, Inc., 1972.

Meinig, Donald W. *The Great Columbia Plain.* Seattle: University of Washington Press, 1968.

Meyers, Jay Arthur. *Captains of All These Men of Death.* St. Louis, Missouri: Warren H. Green, 1977.

Miller, Jay, ed. *Mourning Dove: A Salishan Autobiography.* Lincoln: University of Nebraska Press, 1990.

Moyers, Bill, ed. *Healing and the Mind.* New York: Doubleday, 1993.

Nash, Gary. *Red, White, and Black: The Peoples of Early America.* Englewood Cliffs, New Jersey: Prentice-Hall, 1974.

Nashone. *Grandmother Stories of the Northwest.* Newcastle, California: Sierra Oaks Publishing Company, 1987.

Newell, Colin. *Methods and Models in Demography.* London: Belhaven Press, 1988.

Oliphant, J. Orin. *On the Cattle Ranges of the Oregon Country.* Seattle: University of Washington Press, 1968.

Oregon Improvement Company. *Eastern Washington Territory and Oregon.* Portland: Oregon Improvement Company, 1881.

Ortiz, Alfonso, ed. *Southwest.* Washington, D. C.: Smithsonian Institution Press, 1983.

Pennington, James E., ed. *Respiratory Infections: Diagnosis and Management.* New York: Raven Press, 1983.

Philp, Kenneth R. *John Collier's Crusade for Indian Reform, 1920-1954.* Tucson: University of Arizona Press, 1972.

Preston, Samuel and Michael R. Haines. *Fatal Years: Child Mortality in Late Nineteenth-Century America.* Princeton, New Jersey: Princeton University Press, 1991.

Prucha, Francis Paul. *American Indian Policy in Crisis: Christian Reformers and the Indian, 1865-1900.* Norman: University of Oklahma Press, 1976.

_____. *Indian Policy in the United States.* Lincoln: University of Nebraska Press, 1981.

Ramenofsky, Ann F. *Vectors of Death.* Albuquerque: University of New Mexico Press, 1987.

Ray, Verne F. *Cultural Relations in the Plateau of Northwestern America.* Los Angeles: Southwest Museum, 1939.

Reichwein, Jeffrey C. *Emergence of Native American Nationalism in the Columbia Plateau.* New York: Garland Publishing Company, 1990.

Relander, Click. *Drummers and Dreamers.* Caldwell, Idaho: The Caxton Printers, Ltd., 1956.

_____. *Strangers on the Land.* Yakima, Washington: Franklin Press, 1962.

_____ *The Yakimas: Treaty Centennial.* Yakima, Washington: Republic Press, 1955.

Richards, Kent. *Isaac I. Stevens: Young Man in a Hurry.* Provo, Utah: Brigham Young University Press, 1979. Reprinted by Washington State University Press, 1993

Rollins, Phillip A., ed. *The Discovery of the Oregon Trail.* New York: Charles Scribner's Sons, 1935.

Ronda, James P. *Lewis and Clark Among the Indians.* Lincoln: University of Nebraska Press, 1984.

Ruby, Robert H. and John A. Brown. *A Guide to the Indian Tribes of the Pacific Northwest.* Norman: University of Oklahoma Press, 1986.

_____. *Dreamer-Prophets of the Columbia Plateau: Smohalla and Skolaskin.* Norman: University of Oklahoma Press, 1989.

_____. *Indians of the Pacific Northwest.* Norman: University of Oklahoma Press, 1982.

_____. *John Slocum and the Indian Shaker Church*. Norman: University of Oklahoma Press, 1996

_____. *The Cayuse Indians: Imperial Tribesmen of Old Oregon*. Norman: University of Oklahoma Press, 1972.

Schuster, Helen H. *The Yakima*. New York: Chelsea House Publishers, 1990.

_____. *The Yakimas: A Critical Bibliography*. Bloomington: Indiana University Press, 1982.

Shryock, Henry S., Jacob S. Siegel, and Associates with Condensed Edition by Edward G. Stockwell. *The Methods and Materials of Demography*. San Diego: Academic Press, 1976.

Shryock, Richard Harrison. *National Tuberculosis Association, 1904-1954*. New York: National Tuberculosis Association, 1957.

Simpson, Howard. *Invisible Armies*. Indianapolis: Bobbs-Merrill, 1980.

Sleisenger, Marvin H. and John S. Fordham, eds. *Gastrointestinal Disease*. Philadelphia: W. B. Saunders, 1989.

Smith, F. B. *The Retreat of Tuberculosis, 1850-1950*. London: Croom Helm, 1988.

Snipp, C. M. *American Indians: The First of this Land*. New York: Russell- Sage Foundation, 1987.

Spier, Leslie. "The Prophet Dance of the Northwest and Its Derivatives: The Source of the Ghost Dance, " *General Series in Anthropology*. Menasha, Wisconsin: George Banta Publishing Co., 1953.

_____. "Tribal Distribution in Washington," *General Series in Anthropology*. Menasha, Wisconsin: George Banta Publishing Co., 1936.

Spink, Wesley W. *Infectious Diseases: Prevention and Treatment in the Nineteenth and Twentieth Centuries*. Minneapolis: University of Minnesota Press, 1978.

Splawn, A. J. *Ka-mi-akin, Last Hero of the Yakimas*. Portland, Oregon: Stationary and Printing Company, 1917.

Stearn, E. Wagner, and Allen E. *The Effect of Smallpox on the Destiny of the Amerindian*. Boston: Bruce Humphries, Inc., 1945.

Swanton, John R. *Indian Tribes of North America*. Washington, D. C.: Government Printing Office, 1952.

Teller, Michael. *The Tuberculosis Movement: A Public Health Campaign in the Progressive Era.* New York: Greenwood Press, 1988.

Thornton, Russell. *American Indian Holocaust and Survival: A Population History Since 1492.* Norman: University of Oklahoma Press, 1978.

Trafzer, Clifford E. and Richard D. Scheuerman. *Renegade Tribe: The Palouse Indians and the Invasion of the Inland Pacific Northwest.* Pullman, Washington: Washington University Press, 1986.

Trafzer, Clifford E. ed. *American Indian Identity: Today's Changing Perspectives.* Newcastle, California: Sierra Oaks Publishing Co., 1989.

_____. *American Indian Prophets.* Newcastle, California: Sierra Oaks Publishing Co., 1986.

_____. *Chief Joseph's Allies.* Newcastle, California, Sierra Oaks Publishing Company, 1992

_____. *Indians, Superintendents, and Councils: Northwestern Indian Policy, 1850-1855.* Lanham, Maryland: University Press of America, 1986.

_____. *The Chinook.* New York: Chelsea House Publishers, 1990.

_____. *Yakima, Palouse, Cayuse, Umatilla, Walla Walla, and Wanapum: An Historical Bibliography.* Metuchen, New Jersey: The Scarecrow Press, 1992.

Trevanthan, Wenda R. *Human Birth: An Evolutionary Perspective.* New York: Aldine Le Gruyter, 1987.

Truelove, S. C. *Diseases of the Digestive System.* Oxford: Blackwell Scientific Publications, 1972.

Tyler, Lyman, *A History of Indian Policy.* Washington, D.C.: Government Printing Office, 1973.

Villard, Henry. *The Early History of Transportation in Oregon.* Eugene: University of Oregon Press, 1944.

Vogel, Virgil J. *American Indian Medicine.* Norman: University of Oklahoma Press, 1970.

Waksman, Selman A. *The Conquest of Tuberculosis.* Berkeley: University of California Press, 1964.

Weeks, John R. *Population: An Introduction to Concepts and Issues.* Belmont, California: Wadsworth Publishing Company, 1992.

Williams, J. D. and J. Burnie, eds. *Bacterial Meningitis*. London: Academic Press, 1987.

Zucker, Jeff, Kay Hummel, and Bob Hogfoss. *Oregon Indians: Culture, History, and Current Affairs, An Atlas and Introduction*. Portland: Oregon Historical Society, 1983.

Articles and Chapters

Alter, George. "Infant and Child Mortality in the United States and Canada," paper presented at "La Mortalite des Enfants dans le passe," International Union for the Scientific Study of Population.

Basso, Keith H. "Western Apache." *Southwest*. Washington, D. C.: Smithsonian Institution Press, 1983.

Boyd, Robert T. "Pacific Northwest Measles Epidemic, 1847-1848." *Oregon Historical Quarterly* 95 (1994): 6-47.

Bischoff, William N. "The Yakima Indian War, 1855-56, A Problem in Research." *Pacific Northwest Quarterly* 41 (1950): 162-169.

_____. "Yakima Campaign of 1856," *Mid-America* 31 (1949): 163-208.

Bosch, F. Xavier, et al. "Male Sexual Behavior and Human Papilloma-Virus DNA: Key Risk Factors for Cervical Cancer in Spain." *Journal of the National Cancer Institute* 88 (1996): 1060-1075.

Buechner, Helmutt K. "Some Biotic Changes in the State of Washington, Particularly During the Century 1853-1953." *Research Studies of the State College of Washington* 21 (1953): 154-192.

Buikstra, Jane E., ed. "Prehistoric Tuberculosis in the Americas." *Scientific Papers*, No. 5. Evanston, Illinois: Northwestern University Archaelogical Program, 1981.

Campbell, Gregory R. "The Changing Dimensions of Native American Health: A Critical Understanding of Contemporary Native American Health Issues." *American Indian Culture and Research Journal* 13 (1989): 1- 20.

_____. "The Political Epidemiology of Infant Mortality: A Crisis among Montana American Indians." *American Indian Culture and Research Journal* 13 (1989): 105-148.

Carmichael, Ann G. "Infection, Hidden Hunger, and History." *Journal of Interdiscipinary History* 14 (1983): 249-264.

Carr, Barbara A., and Eun Sul Lee. "Navajo Tribal Mortality: A Life Table Analysis of the Leading Cause of Death." *Social Biology* 25 (1978): 279-287.

Castillo, Edward D. "The Impact of Euro-American Exploration and Settlement." *California.* Washington, D. C.: Smithsonian Institution Press, 1978, pp. 99-127.

Clark, Ella. "George Gibbs' Account of Indian Mythology in Oregon and Washington Territories." *Oregon Historical Quarterly* 56 (1955- 1956): 293-325 and 57 (1955-1956): 125-167.

Coale, George L. "Notes on the Guardian Spirit Concept Among the Nez Perce." *National Archives of Ethnography* 48 (1958).

Coan, C. F. "The Adoption of the Reservation Policy in the Pacific Northwest, 1853-1855." *Oregon Historical Quarterly* 23 (1922): 1-38.

_____. "The First Stage of the Federal Indian Policy in the Pacific Northwest." *Oregon Historical Quarterly* 22 (1921): 46-89.

Colton, J. S. "A Report on the Range Conditions of Central Washington." *Washington State Agricultural College Experiment Station Bulletin* 60 (1904): 5-21.

Cook, Shelburne. F. "The Epidemic of 1830-33 in California and Oregon." *University of California Publications in American Archaeology and Ethnology* 43 (1955): 303-326.

_____. "Population Trends Among the California Mission Indians. *Ibero-Americana* 17, University of California Press, 1940.

Culverwell, Albert. "Stronghold in the Yakima Country: Fort Simcoe and the Indian War, 1856-59." *Pacific Northwest Quarterly* 46 (1955): 46-51.

DeLien, H. and J. Nixon Hadley. "How to Recognize an Indian Health Problem." *Human Organization* (1952): 29-33.

Deutsch, Herman J. "Indian and White in the Inland Empire: The Contest for the Land, 1880-1912." *Pacific Northwest Quarterly* 47 (1956): 44-51.

Dickinson, John A. "The Pre-Contact Huron Population: A Re-Appraisal." *Ontario History* 72 (1980), 173-179.

Dobyns, Henry F. "Estimating Aboriginal American Population: An Appraisal of Techniques with a New Hemisphere Estimate." *Current Anthropology* 7 (1966), 395-416.

_____. "Tribalism Today: An Anthropological Perspective on Reservation Enclaves and Urban Pan-Indians." Paper presented at First Annual Conference on Problems and Issues Concerning American Indians Today. The Newberry Library, 1978.

Douglas, Jesse S. "Origins of the Population in Oregon in 1850." *Pacific Northwest Quarterly* 41 (1950): 95-108.

Emerson, Haven. "Morbidity of the American Indians." *Science* 63, (1926): 229-231.

Hadley, J. Nixon. "Demography of the American Indians." *Annals of the American Academy of Political and Social Science* 311 (1957): 23-30.

Haines, Francis. "Problems of Indian Policy." *Pacific Northwest Quarterly* 41 (1950): 203-212.

_____. "The Northward Spread of Horses Among the Plains Indians." *American Anthropologist* 40 (1938): 429-437.

Hilgard, E. W. "The Yakima and the Clickitat Regions," *The Northwest* 2 (1884): 1-12.

Hill, Charles A., Jr., and Mozart I. Spector. "Natality and Mortality of American Indians Compared with United States Whites and Nonwhites." *Health Reports* 86, (1971): 229-246.

Hoaglin, Lester L., Jr. and Herbert C. Taylor, Jr. "The Intermittent Fever Epidemic of the 1830's on the Lower Columbia River." *Ethnohistory* 2 (1962): 160-178.

Hrdlicka, Ales. "Tuberculosis Among Certain Indian Tribes in the United States." *Annual Report of the Bureau of American Ethnography* 42. Washington, D. C.: Smithsonian Institution, 1909, pp. 1-43.

Jacobs, Melville. "A Sketch of Northern Sahaptin Grammar," *University of Washington Publications in Anthropology* 4 (1931): 83-292.

Johansson, S. Ryan. "Food For Thought: Rhetoric and Reality in Modern Mortality History." *Historical Methods* 27 (1994): 101-125.

Joralemon, Donald. "New World Depopulation and the Case of Disease." *Journal of Anthropological Research* 38 (1982): 108-127

Justice, James W. "Twenty Years of Diabetes on the Warm Springs Reservation, Oregon." *American Indian Culture and Research Journal* 13 (1989): 49-81.

Konlande, J. R. and J. R. K. Robson. "The Nutritive Value of Cooked Camas as Consumed by Flathead Indians." *Ecology of Food and Nutrition* 2 (1972): 193-195.

Lee, M., R. Roburn, and A. Carrow. "Nutritional Studies of British Columbian Indians." *Canadian Journal of Public Health* 62 (1971): 285-296.

McKeown, Thomas. "Food, Infection, and Population." *Journal of Interdisciplinary History* 14 (1983): 227-247.

Merrit, Edgar B. "Health Conditions Among Indians." *Redman* (1914): 347- 350.

Morse, Dan. "Prehistoric Tuberculosis in America," *American Review of Respiratory Diseases* 83 (1961): 489-504.

Neel, James V. "Diabetes Mellitus: A 'Thrifty' Genotype Rendered Detrimental by 'Progress.'" *American Journal of Human Genetics* 14 1962): 353-362.

Nelson, Denys. "Yakima Days." *Washington Historical Quarterly* 19 (1928): 45-51, 117-133, 181-192.

Newman, Marshall T. "Aboriginal New World Epidemiology and Medical Care, and the Impact of the Old World Disease Imports."*American Journal of Physical Anthropology* 45 (1976): 667-672.

Norton, Helen J. and Steven J. Gill. "The Ethnobotanical Imperative: A Consideration of Obligations, Implications, and Methodology." *Northwest Anthropological Research Notes* 15 (1981): 117-187.

Oliphant, J. Orin. "Encroachment of Cattlemen on Indian Reservations in the Pacific Northwest, 1870-1890." *Agricultural History* 24 (1950): 42-58.

_____. "Some Neglected Aspects of the History of the Pacific Northwest." *Pacific Northwest Quarterly* 61 (1970): 1-9.

Omran, Abdel R. "Epidemiologic Transition in the United States: The Health Factor in Population Change." *Population Bulletin* 32 (1977): 1-42.

Painter, Harry. "New Light on Chief Kamiakin." *Walla Walla Union Bulletin* March 18, 1945.

Popkin, Barry M. "Nutritional Patterns and Transitions." *Population and Development Review* 19 (1993): 138-157.

Raviglione, Mario, Dixie Snider, and Arata Kochi. "Global Epidemiology of Tuberculosis." *Journal of the American Medical Association* 18 (1995): 220-226.

Ray, Verne E. "Native Villages and Groupings of the Columbia Basin." *Pacific Northwest Quarterly* 27 (1936): 99-152.

_____. "The Bluejay Character in the Plateau Spirit Dance." *American Anthropologist* 39 (1937): 593-601.

_____. "Tribal Distribution in Eastern Oregon and Adjacent Regions." *American Anthropologist* 40 (1938): 384-415.

Richards, Kent. "Issac Stevens and Federal Military Power in Washington Territory." *Pacific Northwest Quarterly* 63 (1972): 81-86.

Rosen, Laurence S. and Kurt Gorwitz. "New Attention to American Indians." *American Demographics* 2 (1980): 18-25.

Roth, Eric Abella. "Demography and Computer Simulation in Historic Village Population Reconstruction." *Journal of Anthropological Research* 3 (1981):279-301.

Schneider, Keith. "Nuclear Complex Threatens Indians." *New York Times*, National Edition, September 3, 1990.

Scott, Leslie M. "Indian Disease as Aids to Pacific Northwest Settlement." *Oregon Historical Quarterly* 19 (1928): 99-107.

Siegel, Jacob S. "Estimates of Coverage of the Population by Sex, Race, and Age in the 1970 Census." *Demography* 11 (1974): 1-23.

Slagle, Al Logan. "Tolowa Indian Shakers and the Role of Prophecy at Smith River, California." *American Indian Prophets*. Newcastle, California: Sierra Oaks Publishing Company, 1981.

Stanley, Sam, and Robert K. Thomas. "Current Demographic and Social Trends Among North American Indians." *Annals of the American Academy of Political and Social Science* 436 (1978): 111-120.

Stearn, E. Wagner, and Allen E. Stearn. "Smallpox Immunization of the Amerindian." *Bulletin of the History of Medicine* 13 (1943):601-613.

Taylor, Herbert C., Jr., and Lester L. Hoaglin. "The 'Intermittent Fever.' Epidemic of the 1830s on the Lower Columbia River." *Ethnohistory* 9, (1962):160-178.

Thornton, Russell. "American Indian Historical Demography: A Review Essay with Suggestions for Future Research." *American Indian Culture and Research Journal* 3 (1979): 69-74

____and Joan Marsh-Thornton. "Estimating Prehistoric American Indian Population Size for United States Area: Implications of the Nineteenth Century Population Decline and Nadir." *American Journal of Physical Anthropology* 55 (1981): 47-53.

Trafzer, Clifford E. "Horses, Cattle, Buggies, Hacks: Purchases by Yakima Indian Women, 1909-1912." In , *Negotiators of Change: Historical Perspectives on Native American Women.* Nancy Shoemaker, ed. New York: Routledge, 1995, pp. 176-192.

Trafzer, Clifford E., and Margery Ann Beach. "Smohalla, the Washani, and Religion as a Factor in Northwestern Indian History." *American Indian Quarterly* 9 (1985): 309-324.

Wagner, Carruth J., and Erwin S. Rabeau. "Indian Poverty and Indian Health." *United States Department of Health, Education, and Welfare Indicators* (1964): xxiv-xliv.

Watkins, Susan Cott and Etienne van de Walle. "Nutrition, Mortality, and Population Size: Malthus' Court of Last Resort." *Journal of Interdisciplinary History* 14 (1983): 205-226.

Weiss, K. M., and P.E. Smouse. "The Demographic Stability of Small Human Populations," In *The Demographic Evolution of Human Populations.* London: Academic Press, 1976.

Whitner, R. L., "Grant's Indian Peace Policy on the Yakima Reservation, 1870-1882,"*Pacific Northwest Quarterly* 50 (1959): 135-142.

INDEX

accidents: as cause of death, 8, 70, 88, 93, 172, 196; in children age two to six, 170-71; in children of one year, 167, 172; children's death from, 150, 168-173, 183n. 53; crude death rates from, 135-36, 137-38, 200, 204; death rate comparisons, 135-38, 143, 175, 194; and gender, 167, 170, 174-75, 177, 194, 195

accidents, automobile: as cause of death, 102, , 121n. 79, 137-38, 150; crude death rates from, 135-38; death rate from, 100, 143; and gender, 175

accidents, miscellaneous: as cause of death, 93, 100-101, 135-36, 148-49, 196; in children, 167; death rate from, 133

African-Americans: and accidents, 135, 136; and cancer, 139-40; death rate comparisons, 86, 93, 123, 137; and heart disease, 133; infant mortality, 94; and miscellaneous causes of death, 133, 137, 138, 141, 142; mortality, 69, 71, 86, 93, 94; and pneumonia, 130, 131, 132; and tuberculosis, 128, 129, 193

age at death data, 15, 79, 86, 89-90

agents. *See* Indian Agents

Age of Degeneration and Man-Made Diseases, 2, 3, 69, 70-71

Age of Pestilence and Famine, 2-3, 69-70, 73, 76, 144; death data from, 91,

199; end of, 151, 188; and reservations, 187

Age of Receding Pandemics, 2, 3, 69-70, 151, 188; death data from, 199

Alaskan Natives, 164

alcohol, 76, 106; as cause of death, 71, 90, 102, 175, 178, 205; and gender, 177, 178, 195

animal spirits, 47

Annual Reports of the Commissioner of Indian Affairs, 14

anthropology, 1

antibiotics, 88, 96, 97, 101, 129; scarcity of, 146, 150

Apache People, 126

arthritis, 92

autopsies, 7, 121n. 86, 140, 159, 178

Benson, Todd, 116n. 26

birthrate: pre-white contact, 72; Yakama, 11, 15

Birth Registers, 1, 15, 31, 161, 162, 188

blood quantum data, 78, 86, 110, 111-12, 194

Bolon, Andrew Jackson, 29

Boyd, Robert, 103, 126

Broncheau, Evelyn, 199

bronchitis, 91

Brookings Institute, 81

Buchanen, James, 30, 108

buffalo, 27, 33, 198

Bureau of Indian Affairs: Health Division, 45, 164

burials, 48-57, 64-65n. 73

Campbell, Gregory R., 203

cancer, 2; as cause of death, 7, 93, 104, 121n. 86, 143; crude death rate from, 200; death rate comparisons, 139-40, 143, 175-76, 194, 202, 204; and diet, 139-40; and gender, 90, 104, 140, 175-76, 177, 194, 195; rise of, 3, 70, 88. *See also* autopsies; smoking

canoes, 52

cardiovascular disease. *See* heart disease

Carmichael, Ann G., 3-4

Carr, Donald M., 35, 46, 124-25, 139, 155-56

Cascade People, 26

Catholic church, 28

cause of death: in censuses, 76-77; changes in primary, 88, 96, 191, 199; for children under six, 90, 98, 146-51; clinical, 7-8, 16-17, 123, 141, 142, 191-93; data quality, 123, 144; from Death Certificates, 67-112, 191, 196; 1888 to 1964, 123, 130, 132, 135-36, 143, 145, 173; fetal, 143-46, 154-58; and gender, 90, 173-79; infant and child, 143, 146-51, 154, 158-61; medical, 7, 123, 141, 142; minor, 92; most frequent, 123-24, 128, 131, 132, 135, 173; native beliefs about, 39-42, 57, 191-93; physical, 40; pollution as, 75, 176, 195-96; pre-European contact, 72, 76, 88; primary, 12, 98, 100, 123, 128-37, 141-45, 171; rankings, 93; and rattlesnake power, 39, 40, 41; reporting accuracy, 39-42, 82-83, 92; secondary, 91, 92-93, 95,

96, 100; SIDS, 150, 184n. 59; by spirit sickness, 37, 39, 40-42, 191-92; suffocation, 150; unknown, 82, 83, 91-92, 96; as a variable, 15, 91-107; white contact and, 39-42; white settlement and, 69, 72, 74, 76, 88. *See also* accidents; alcohol; cancer; coding; diabetes; gastrointestinal disorders; gender; heart disease; influenza; meningitis; murder; pneumonia; smallpox; statistical analysis; suicide; tuberculosis; variables

cause of death data, 91-107. *See also* statistical analysis

Cayuse People, 26, 91, 110, 151

Cayuse War (1848), 41, 151

cemeteries, 51, 52

census: death data from, 76-77, 163; of 1900, 163-64; "non-whites" category on, 157; reservation, 15, 30-31, 78-79; Yakama, 12, 15, 31, 85

chicken pox, 76

chiefs, "head", 33. *See also under specific names*

children. *See* cause of death; mortality

cholera, 2

Christianity, 84; and Yakama conversion, 5, 28, 38, 44, 187, 189

Cíkik (village), 26

cis, 47-48, 52

Clark, William, 2, 27, 69. *See also* Lewis and Clark Expedition

Clayman, Charles B., 98

Coale-Demeny model life tables, 72

coding, cause-of-death data, 92-94, 100, 121n. 79, 150; for age at death, 89; for blood quamtum, 112; numeric, 91; for place, 108; for tribe, 109

coffins, 52

colds, 92

"cold sickness". *See* influenza

Collier, John, 83, 87

Colville Reservation, 16, 17, 61n. 27

communications: disease, and, 126, 129; telephone, 47, 84

comparisons. *See* cause of death; crude death rate; death rate; population comparisons; statistical analysis

consumption. *See* tuberculosis

correspondence. *See* letterbooks

Covington, Corky, 199

Coyote (Spilyay), 24-25, 27, 59n. 4

Crow Reservation, 15

crude death rates, 9, 10; comparisons, 93, 117n. 33, 123, 124, 128-29, 144; decline of, 197; population comparisons of, 31, 72, 123-79, 193-96, 200; reservation, 144, 196. *See also under specific names*

culture, loss of, 187-192. *See also* Indian agents; religion; reservation; white settlement; Yakima People

dams, 115n. 17, 173, 197

Dance of the Dead, 43

death: beliefs, 47-57; as a natural "law", 25; unreported, 82-85; in Yakama culture, 38, 39-40, 42, 46-57. *See also* cause of death; crude death rates; Death Certificates; death rate; Death Registers; death statistics; mortality; spirit sickness

Death Certificates, 1, 12-15, 87, 139, 188, 195; accuracy of, 31, 39, 57, 69, 158, 162; data quality in, 78, 82-84, 89, 123, 144; decline in 1940s, 88-89; and epidemiological transitions, 69-71, 72, 76; history, 190; as information sources, 13-15, 68, 85-86, 188-91; and mortality, 6-7; and population comparisons, 69, 86, 90, 93-94; statistical analysis of deaths from, 86-112; variables in, 86-112; warnings of, 47; Yakama, 68-71, 76-112, 191. *See also* cause of death; death

rate; death statistics; Meriam, Lewis; variables

death data. *See* death statistics

death-over-time studies, 68-69, 86

death rate, 8, 9, 31; decline in, 87-89, 96; intervals, 123; population comparisons, 123-79, 193-95, 203; statistics, 7, 39, 193. *See also* crude death rate; population comparisons

Death Registers, 1, 68, 78, 161; accuracy of, 31, 69; history of, 12-13, 15, 188, 190; and mortality data, 6, 85

death statistics, 7; accuracy of, 39-40, 78; analysis of, 86-112; bases, 190; as information source, 191; recording history 190-93; variables, 78, 86-112. *See also* age at death; blood quantum; cause of death; coding; gender of deceased; place of death; tribal affiliation; ward; year of death

De Lien, H., 10, 83

Department of Health and Human Services, 45, 164

Department of Health, Education, and Welfare, 45, 164

Department of the Interior, 164

depression: and health, 9, 70, 87; social, 5, 189, 206

DeWitt, John, 12

diabetes: 71, 88, 105, 106, 201-204; epidemics, 2

diet: changes in, 127, 189, 198-99; and disease, 80, 94, 97, 99, 100, 130; fiber and, 134; fat composition of, 3, 134, 140; Popkin's theories on, 3; programs, 197. *See* food; nutrition; white settlement

diphtheria, 92

discrimination: by   government institutions, 28-31; by whites, 28-29

disease: Columbia Plateau history of, 10-12, 30, 39, 69-70, 76, 198-99, 206; and depression, 9, 70, 87; epidemics, 2, 69, 77, 79; European, 69, 76; and food, 3-4, 71, 126; and health programs, 5, 135; immunity, 72; infectious, 126. 198; and language barriers, 126, 129; man-made, 2; overview of, 2, 6, 70; spread of, 6, 30, 53-54, 126, 187-90; and state of mind, 125; and white contact, 31, 39-43, 71, 126; "white man's", 30, 39-41, 46, 76, 172. *See also under specific names*; cause of death; diet; diseases; epidemics; epidemiological transition; health; medicine; mortality; Yakama

diseases. *See under specific names*

doctors. *See* medicine men

drug use, 205

DuBois, Cora, 43

Dubos, Jean and René, 125-26, 129, 160

education: disease prevention, 124, 128-29, 135, 136; hygiene, 46

elders: deaths of, 85, 103; funeral role of, 53; healing role of, 36-37, 40, 46, 75, 156, 192; George, 24; Nelson, 17; Smartlowit, 27

Encyclopedia of Medicine, 98

Entiat People, 110

environment and mortality, 4, 8-11. *See also* health; pollution; white settlement

epidemics, 11, 30, 40-41, 43, 81, 202; white contact, 69, 77, 79, 91. *See also under specific names;* Age of Degeneration and Man-Made Diseases; Age of Pestilence and Famine; Age of Receding Pandemics

epidemiological transition, 4, 68-72, 144, 187, 204, 205-206; influences on, 1-3, 144, 198; overlapping periods of, 2-3, 69-71, 72, 76, 151, 188; post-World War II, 198-207. *See also* epidemics; nutrition; Omran, Abdel R.

epilepsy, 92

Estep, Evan W., 38, 39

eye ailments, 71, 76

faith. *See* Wáshani; Wáshat

farming, 4

Fatal Years: Child Mortality in Late Nineteenth-Century America, 4

Feather religion, 44, 45, 189

fertility rate, 72

fetal death. *See* cause of death; mortality

Fetal Years (Preston and Haines), 163

fevers, 2, 11, 69, 91

field matrons. *See* Sprague, Esther M.

Fleming, Alexander, 150

food: destruction of native, 4-5, 132-33, 197-98; and mortality, 4-5; refined, 71, 88, 94, 132, 198-99, 202, 203-204; and spirituality, 25, 202. *See also* diet; nutrition; root gathering

Fort Simcoe, 29, 45, 46, 84, 108

Fort Vancouver, 41

funding and health programs, 188. *See also* health

funerals, 48-57, 64n. 73

gall bladder disease, 202

Garza, Pam, 199

gastrointestinal disorders, 8, 11, 95; as cause of death, 70, 88, 93, 101-102, 136-37, 199; in children, 146-47, 159, 171; in children at age one, 165-67; in children age two to six, 169-70; death rate comparison of, 136-37, 166-67, 175; decline of, 87, 136, 137; and gender, 159, 166, 170, 175, 177; in infants, 159

gender: and cancer, 104, 140, 175, 177; and cause of death, 173-79, 194; and data comparisons, 176-79; in death data, 15, 78, 79, 86, 90, 173-79, 195; and infant deaths, 155, 158-61

General Allotment Act, 78-79

George, Andrew, 24, 64n. 73

ghosts, 47-48, 52

give-away ceremony, 53, 54

gold rush, 29

government: health actions, 81-83; Indian policies and disease, 73, 126-27; wards, 111-12. *See also* Department of Health and Human Services; health; Indian Agents; Office of Indian Affairs

grave desecration, 57, 65n. 84

Griffith, Dr. 55

Guardian Spirit Complex (Spier), 32

Guie, Dean, 16

Guie, Geraldine, 16

Hadley, J. Nixon, 10, 83

Haines, Michael R., 4, 71, 88, 163

Hanford Nuclear Plant. *See* pollution

Harrah, Washington, 108

hawluk, 47-48

health: decline, 29-30, 74-77; funding, 188; and housing, 74, 75, 80, 94; improvement, 199; monitoring, 190-91; relationship to state of mind, 8-9; services, 2, 188, 196. *See also* disease; epidemics; government; public health

Health & Hospitalization Records and Reports, 1912-1940, 155

heart disease, 88; after WW II, 132; as cause of death, 3, 8, 95, 98-100, 123, 132, 174; causes of, 132-35; in children, 146, 150, 161, 171; crude death rates from, 132, 133, 177, 200; death rate comparisons, 132-35, 143, 160-61, 181n. 26, 194, 204; and gender, 160, 176; in infants, 160-61; pre-white contact, 76; and refined foods, 71, 88, 94, 132; rise of, 2, 3, 70, 143; treatment, 75. *See also* population comparisons

herbology, 40, 75

high blood pressure, 202. *See also* heart disease

Historical Statistics of the United States: Colonial Times to 1970, 9

Ho Chunk, 53-54

Hogfoss, Bob, 11

Holm, Kirsten, 13

homesteads, native, 13-14, 77

homicide. *See* murder

horses, 25, 26, 27, 59n. 8

Horst, Jim, 199

hospitals: at Toppenish, 35, 47, 84, 108, 197; lack of, 46, 75, 125, 188

housing: changes, 189; and health, 74-75, 80, 84, 97, 127, 129, 130; improved, 12; substandard, 6, 9, 75, 94, 189; tipi, 27, 74, 94, 127, 189

Hoxie, Frederick, 15

Humishuma (Mourning Dove), 16-17, 61n. 27

Hummel, Kay, 11

Hunn, Eugene S., 27, 40, 47; on death rates, 88, 158; on diabetes, 202, 203; on Native history, 10-11; on reservations, 8

Hunt, Jake, 44

Husum (village), 44

hygiene, 46, 74-75, 94, 189; education, 124, 128-29, 135, 136

Idaho, 27, 46

illness, causes of, 40

Indian Agents, 30, 31, 35; attitudes of, 40, 41-42, 84, 155, 192; Bolon, 29; Carr, 35, 46, 124-25, 139, 155-56; destructive activities of, 188-89; Estep, 38, 39; recordkeeping of, 84, 117n. 33, 188, 190

Indian Health Service, 196-97

Indian Homestead Act, 13. *See also* homesteads

Indian Medical Services, 45

Indian New Deal, 2

industrial exposure, 2, 3

infant mortality. *See* mortality

influenza, 2, 3, 11, 75, 199; as cause of death, 81, 91, 93, 95, 102-103, 138-39; in children of one year, 168; death rate comparison, 138-39, 175, 193, 194-95; epidemics, 41, 43, 91, 103, 138-39, 167-68; and gender, 175, 177; and white settlement, 69, 70, 71, 76, 77

Institute of Government Research, 81

Jim, Charlie, 51, 52

Jim, Fishhook, 51-52

Jim, Mary, 51, 52, 56

Johansson, S. Ryan, 4

John, Sharon, 199

Justice, James W., 203-204

Justis, Joyce, 67

Kamiakin (Chief), 29, 33-34, 43; grave of, 57, 65n. 84

Kamoshnite, 33

Kittitas People (Upper Yakama), 27

Klickitat People, 14, 26, 44, 69, 188

Kober, George M., 79

Koch, Robert, 125

Koenig, Margaret W., 53

Kofford, Linda, 199

Kotiahkan, 43, 44

Lament of the Dead ceremony, 56

language: barriers and disease, 126, 129; Chinook, 14, 30; destruction, 155; English, 5; families, 72, 110; Sahaptin, 27, 30; Salish, 30, 58n. 1, 61n. 27; Yakama, 5, 30

"laws" in Yakama spirituality, 24-25

letterbooks, 67, 77, 155

Lewis, Meriwether, 2, 27, 69. *See also* Lewis and Clark Expedition

Lewis and Clark Expedition (1805), 27, 41, 69

life expectancy, 72

malaria, 11, 69, 71; epidemics, 40, 41, 91, 103

malnutrition, 146, 147, 148

McKeown, Thomas, 3, 4

McWhorter, Lucullus V., 55, 58n. 1

measles, 2, 11, 30, 75, 100, 150-51; epidemics, 41, 43, 69, 77, 91, 202; pre-white contact, 40

medicine: impediments to getting, 46-47, 188; prenatal care, 155-56; rattlesnake, 16; traditional native, 30, 40, 45. *See also* disease; medicine man; spirituality

medicine men, and women, (twati), 33, 34-40, 41, 45, 46; affected by reservations, 156; ineffectual with new diseases, 75-76, 192; influence and power of, 34-39; power misuse by, 37-39; suppression of, 35, 38

meningitis, 90, 95, 149-50, 183n. 56; in children, 170, 172; and gender, 170, 177-78, 195

Meninick (chief), 38, 39

Meriam, Lewis, 81-83

Meriam Report, The, 81-83, 87, 157

missionaries, 28, 38, 43, 151; and burials, 52

"modernization", 3, 71, 99, 198, 199

Modern Rise of Population, The (McKeown), 4

Montana, 27, 29

Moran, John, 199

mortality: Afro-American, 69, 71, 86, 93, 94; child, 8, 31, 71, 79, 85, 88,

163; by age-group, 204-205; of children age two to six, 168-71; of children of one year, 165-68; children under six, 8, 90, 98, 146-51; comparisons, 71, 90, 123-78, 193-94, 199-207; declines, 2, 88, 163; and environment, 4, 8-11; fetal, 8, 9, 10, 93, 144-46, 156-58; and food, 4; and gender, 90, 165, 166, 169, 173-79; incomplete data on, 79, 85; increases, 4, 162; infant, 8, 9, 31, 71, 89-90, 93-94, 144, 158-65; influences on, 4-5; of Native Americans, 9-11; patterns, 2-3, 7-8, 9, 205; rate predictability, 72; report, 199-203; on reservation, 71; reservation vs. urban, 8; statistics, 8, 10, 190, 203; in transition eras, 144; Yakama, 2-5, 9-13. *See also* cause of death; crude death rate; epidemics; statistical analysis

Mourning Dove, 16-17, 61n. 27

mourning rituals, 48, 49-57, 85

Moxee City, Washington, 108

mumps, 149

murder, 71, 178, 179, 199, 200, 201; and age-groups, 205

Nash, Gary, 14

Nason, Ida, 37

National Archives, Pacific Northwest Region, 7, 67, 68, 77-78, 195

National Tuberculosis Association, 79, 80, 81

Neel, James, 203

Nelson, Mary, 17

New Deal (Indian), 83, 128, 150

Nez Perce People, 42, 46, 110

1991 Mortality Report, 199-203

Nisqually People, 44, 110

"non-whites", 94, 104, 157, 158, 162, 164

nutrition: decline and reservations, 156; and mortality, 3-4, 8-11; programs, 197; transitions in, 144, 187, 197-99, 202, 203, 206. *See also* diet; food; epidemiological transition

Office of Indian Affairs: and disease spread, 73, 75, 76; and farm changes, 74; and fetal deaths, 155; and funeral changes, 52; and health decline, 74-75, 188; health division, 151-52, 172, 196; health education programs of, 5-6, 82, 124, 128-29, 139, 155; record keeping of, 12, 68, 78-79, 82-83, 87; reforms in, 87, 139; statistics monitoring by, 190; suppressed spirituality, 35, 42, 45, 46; as Yakama supervisors, 29-30, 31, 188-89

Okanagan People, 110

old age: as cause of death, 93, 107, 141-42; death rate comparisons, 142

Omran, Abdel R., 91; on diet, 99, 178; epidemiological theories of, 1-2, 4, 69, 76

oral literature, 1, 17

Oregon Trail, 28

Oregon Volunteers, 151

Osler, William, 125

Owhi (chief), 29

owl spirit symbology, 47

paláxsiks tradition, 53-55

Palouse People, 14, 24, 26, 30, 69, 151; ceremonies of, 56; prophets of, 42; overview of, 67, 188

parotitis, 91

patkwatana, 47

páyuwi (disease), 40

penicillin. *See* antibiotics

place of death data, 15, 78, 86, 108-109

Plateau Indian War (1855-58), 5, 187

pneumonia, 3, 11; causes, 95, 97, 130; in children, 130, 146, 171; in children age two to six, 169; in children at age one, 165; crude death rate, 130, 131, 193, 200; death rate, 8, 9;

death rate comparisons of, 130-32, 143, 165-68, 193; epidemics, 40, 69, 91; eradication of, 130; and gender, 158, 169, 174, 177; in infants, 158-89; as a leading cause of death, 70, 71, 123, 142-43, 92-93, 97-98, 199; as a main cause of death, 123, 133; spread of, 130; types, 97. *See also* population comparisons

pollution, 75, 176, 195-96

Popkin, Barry, 1, 4, 69; "modernization" theory of, 3, 71, 99, 199

population comparisons: with Death Certificate data, 69, 86, 90, 93-94, 196; of death rates, 123-79, 193-95, 203. *See also* African Americans; crude death rates

population growth, 11, 72, 188, 196, 200, 206

poverty. *See* reservations

power. *See* medicine men; spirits

premature births: as cause of death, 105-107, 122n. 90, 140-41, 172, 199; death rate comparisons, 141, 176, 194; gender of, 176, 177

Preston, Samuel H., 4, 71, 88, 163

Problem of Indian Administration, The (Meriam), 81-83, 87

Progressive Era, 78, 79

prophets, Native, 42-44. *See also* Wáshani

Pswánwapam People, 26, 27, 30, 58n.

public health education, 5-6, 188

Public Health Service, 45, 88, 96, 164

Public Law 83-568 (Transfer Act), 164, 196

Qualchin (chief), 29

Quinault People, 110

rattlesnake medicine, 16, 39, 40, 41, 191

Ray, Verne, 58n. 1

rebirth, 42, 43, 44

reforms in Native affairs, 83, 87, 164; and health, 139, 141

religion: conversion and, 189; Yakama, 23-25, 28, 31-57. *See also* Waptashi; Wáshani; Wáshat religion; Shaker; Yakama

Renegade Tribe: The Palouse Indians and the Invasion of the Inland Pacific Northwest (Trafzer and Scheuerman), 67

reservation(s): caused health decline, 31, 73, 75-76, 80, 84-85, 155; census, 15; changed native lifestyles, 144, 152-53, 156, 173, 187-92; Colville, 16, 17, 61n. 27; Crow, 15; culture on, 191; dangerous life on, 8, 144, 196; and epidemics, 40-41, 95, 126, 144; life as farmers on, 4, 9, 74, 114n. 17, 127; and mortality causes, 71, 144, 151-54; native culture on, 16, 187-92; origins, 73; population, 15; poverty on, 126-27, 130, 151, 172; record keeping on, 12-15; relocation to, 5, 8, 14, 147, 152, 173; Warm Springs, 43, 64n. 73; white culture on, 16, 192, 196. *See also* diet; seasonal rounds; Yakama Reservation

rickets, 92, 178

Ritchie, Brad, 7

rituals. *See* Wáshat religion

Rockefeller, John D., Jr., 81

Roosevelt, Franklin D., 83

root gathering, 4-5; Yakama, 3, 9, 23-26, 30, 127, 132. *See also* food; seasonal rounds

Rosenkrantz, Barbara Gutmann, 94

Salish language, 30, 58n.1, 61n. 27

salmon, 25, 26, 115n. 17, 134, 173, 189

Salo, Wilmar L., 147-48

Sandos, James, 7

sanitariums, 46

sanitation, 2, 6, 75, 80, 97, 130, 188; education, 124, 127-29, 136; improved, 12, 197

scarlatina, 91

scarlet fever epidemic, 41

Schmidt, Karen, 199

Schuster, Helen, 37, 50

scrofula. *See* tuberculosis

seasonal rounds (migratory lifestyle), 9, 25-27, 30, 115n. 17; reservation system ended, 74, 127, 135, 173, 189, 197

Selam, James, 40

senility, 93, 107, 141-42, 176

settlement. *See* white settlement

Shaker Church, 35, 44-45, 189

Shoshoni People, 26, 59n. 8

Showaway (chief), 43

Sioux People, 126

Slocum, John, 44-45

smallpox, 2, 3, 11, 30; epidemics, 40, 41, 43, 91, 202; spread of, 91; and white settlement, 69, 71, 76, 77

Smartlowit, Gilbert, 27

Smohalla (prophet), 42-43

smoking, 99, 104, 132, 134; and cancer, 139, 176

Snyder Act, 45

social history, Yakama, 5, 6, 14, 29, 189, 206. *See also* Yakama

Spier, Leslie, 31-32

Spilyay (Coyote), 24-25, 27, 59n. 4

spirits: Coyote (Spilyay), 24-25, 27, 59n. 4; Guardian, 32; and power, 32-35, 40; tah (tutors), 32-33, 34; warning, 47-48. *See also* medicine man

spirit sickness, 16-17, 36-37; and medicine men, 75, 76; death from, 17, 41-42, 191-92

spiritual beliefs: and death, 21n. 33, 191-92; and food, 25; Guardian Spirit Complex, 32; and illness, 40; and nature, 73; as survival system, 11-12; Yakama, 23-25, 31-57, 59nn. 3-4. *See also* spirits

Spokane, Washington, 108

Spokane People, 110

Sprague, Esther M., 46, 156

standard of living, 2

statistical analysis: age-adjusted, 200-201, 203; cause-of-death rankings, 93; coding for, 89, 90-94, 100, 108, 109, 112, 121n. 79; comparative death data from, 86; data fluctuation in, 86; interval-level variables in, 87, 89; means, 89; modes, 89, 171; moving averages in, 86, 157, 163, 164; nominal variables in, 90, 91, 108, 111; "non-white" category, 157, 158; standard deviation, 89; of Yakama deaths, 86-112, 196

statistical bases, 190

statistics, purpose of, 190-91

Stevens, Isaac Ingalls, 29, 114n. 16

stroke, 2, 90, 107, 195, 200

suicide, 71, 76, 178-79, 199, 200-202, 205

Sunkhaye, 33

Sunnyside, Washington, 108

superstition, 192

Sutherland, Jim, 199

suyapo, 192

sweat lodge, 32, 45, 48

syphilis, 75, 91, 95, 96, 106, 107; in children, 149, 171-72; in infants, 161

Tacoma, Washington, 108

tah (tutelary spirit), 32-33, 34; types, 33, 34, 36-37

tamanwas (power), 34

Tasawick People, 56

tawtnúk (medicine), 40

Teias (chief), 33

telephones, 47

Tenax (chief), 33

Tenino People, 30

Texanap, 36-37

Thompson, David, 27-28

thrush epidemic, 91

tipi, 27, 74, 94, 127, 189

tobacco. *See* smoking

Toppenish (Washington) hospital, 35, 47, 84, 108, 197

traders, 27-28

Transfer Act (1954), 164, 196

transitions. *See* epidemiological transition; nutrition

transportation: as causes of death, 109; funeral, 51; influence on health, 46, 109; lack of as medical impediment, 46-47, 75, 84-85; types, 46

treaties: and health, 5; and hunting rights, 73-74, 114n. 16, 197; and reservations, 13, 29

tribal affiliation data, 30, 69, 78, 86, 108-11

Tsiyiyak, 33,

tuberculosis, 3, 6, 9, 11, 12, 142; age-groups and, 205; as cause of death, 80-81, 91-92, 93, 94-97, 128, 173, 199; causes of, 125; in children, 146-47, 148, 169, 171; in children at age one, 166-67; in children age two to six, 169; consumption, 91, 95-96, 116n. 23; crude death rate, 124, 128, 129, 193; death rate comparisons, 124-30, 142, 159-61, 195; decline of, 2, 87-88, 96, 129, 131, 142, 191; diagnosis of, 94, 125, 129; epidemics, 81, 124, 126, 128-29, 147-48; eradica-tion of, 94, 96-97, 128; funding and, 79; and gender, 160, 166-67, 169, 173, 176-77, 195; importance of, 142; in infants, 159-60; origins of, 126, 147; population comparisons, 124,

148; as primary killer, 12, 93, 173, 183n. 48; record accuracy, 124; scrofula, 6, 80, 116n. 23, 125; spread of, 53-54, 80, 95, 125-30, 146-48; studies of Native American, 53, 79; and white settlement, 69, 70, 71, 80. *See also* epidemics; population com-parisons; sanitariums

Tuberculosis Among the Nebraska Winnebago: a Social Study on an Indian Reservation (Koenig), 53

Turner, Paul A., 79-80

twati. *See* medicine men

typhoid, 2, 71, 91

typhus, 71

ulcers, 2, 3, 11

Umatilla People, 110; prophets, 42

United States Public Health Service, 196

University of Minnesota, 147, 148

variables, eight in death certificate data, 86-112. *See also* age at death data; blood quantum data; cause of death data; gender of deceased data; place of death data; tribal affiliation data; ward data; year of death data

vision quest, 32, 33, 34, 36, 37, 42

vital statistics, 13, 190. *See also* census; death; mortality

Waiilatpu, 151

Waksman, Selman, 96, 147

Walla Walla Council, 74, 114n. 16

Walla Walla People, 26, 29

Walle, Etienne van de, 4

Wallula People, 56

Wanapum People, 14, 26, 42-43, 56, 69, 110

wánpsa (power song), 32

wánpsa (winter sing), 44

Wapato, Washington, 108

Waptailmin (Narrow River People), 58n. 1

Waptashi (Feather religion), 44, 45, 189

ward death data, 86, 111

Warm Springs Reservation, Oregon, 43, 64n. 73, 203-204

wars, 5, 29, 33-34, 41

Wasco People, 26, 30, 69

Wáshani (religion), 31, 45, 49; afterlife in, 42, 44; changes after white contact, 43; and death, 42, 46-57; and funerals, 52; influenced by Christianity, 44; prophets, 33, 42-44; spirits in, 42. *See also* sweat lodge; Yakama

wáshat (dance), 43,

Wáshat (religion), 17, 31, 52, 189

Washington Territory, 28-29

watayíylam (witch), 37

Watkins, Susan Cotts, 4

wátsa (vision quest), 32, 33, 34, 36, 37, 42

Weeks, John R., 72

Wenatchee People, 14, 26

Wenatchi People, 14, 26, 30, 36, 69

Western expansion, 9. *See also* white settlement

white culture: changes brought by, 28-30, 43, 192, 197-99; death data reporting by, 39-40, 42; early contact with, 27-28; life on reservations, 16, 192; settlers, 28, 43. *See also* disease; discrimination; health

"white man's disease", 30, 39-41, 46, 76, 172, 192

White Plague: Tuberculosis, Man, and Society, The (Dubos and Dubos), 125-26, 160

white settlement: changes brought by, 28-30, 172-73, 187-92, 197-99; and

depression, 5, 9, 70, 87; and habitat, 73, 74-75; and native resource loss, 4-5, 9, 70-72, 76, 127, 205. *See also* disease

White Swan, Washington, 108

Whitman, Marcus and Narcissa, 41, 151

whooping cough, 76; in children, 149, 172; in children of one year, 167-68, 172; epidemics, 40, 41, 91; and gender, 167

widower and widow traditions, 53-55

Wilbur, James, 35, 70

Williams, Mrs. Caesar, 54

Winnebago People, 53-54

Wishram People, 26, 30, 69, 188

witchcraft, 16, 32, 37-41, 191, 192

women: as caretakers, 6, 153, 166, 174; as healers, 46, 153; mourning role of, 50; roles changed by reservations, 153, 156, 174; work roles of, 174

Wright, George, 29

Wyoming, 27

xwyáyc (sweat lodge), 32, 45, 48

Yakama, defined, 58n. 1

Yakama Agency, 12, 13, 83, 89, 188

Yakama Indian Agency Papers, 67, 82-83. *See also* Death Certificates

Yakama Indian Health Center, 196-97, 204-205

Yakama People: death effect on, 29, 46-57; fourteen tribes, 26, 30-31, 69, 110, 147, 152, 188; funeral customs, 31-46; health decline, 29-30, 31, 164, 199; land of, 23-24, 59nn. 3-4; Lower, 26, 27, 30, 58n. 1; medicine, 30; overview of, 2-3, 7, 8-9, 23-57, 58n. 1; population changes in, 11, 15-16, 188, 200; prophets, 42-44; religion of, 17, 23-25, 28, 31-57;

seasonal rounds of, 25-27, 30; societal depression in, 29; spirituality of, 23-25, 31-57, 59nn. 3-4; suppression of, 29-31, 35, 45, 46; survival traits of, 11-12, 31; Upper, 26, 27, 30, 58n. 1; and white domination, 29-30, 85. *See also* Birth Registers; cause of death; Death Certificates; Death Registers; disease; epidemiological transitions; health; language; medicine men; mortality; reservation; white culture

Yakama Reservation: boundaries, 108; dangerous life on, 8, 144, 196; and the General Allotment Act, 78-79, 108, 116n. 25; inadequacies, 75, 80, 126-27; mortality study, 1, 3-7, 9, 11-18; origins, 29-30; recordkeeping on, 82-83; resource loss on, 127, 132. *See also* diet; epidemiological transitions; nutrition; reservation; seasonal rounds; white culture; white settlement

Yakama Treaty (1855), 13, 67; broken, 172; described, 8-9, 29, 70, 110; hunting rights restricted, 73-74; 132-33; opposition to, 33

Yakama War (1855-58), 29, 33-34

Yakima: etymology of, 27, 58n. 1; name spelling, 19n. 1

Yakima City, Washington, 108

Yakima County Health Department, 190

Yakima River, 23; habitat, 26-27

Yannaneck, 34

year of death data, 15, 86, 87-89

yellow fever, 91

Zucker, Jeff, 11